Preparing for Birth:

Mothers

Acknowledgements

Andrea Robertson originally wrote this book for Birth International. She wrote the first edition of this book in 1987 through to the fifth edition in 2011. Sadly, in 2015 Andrea died unexpectedly. Jane Palmer has revised this sixth edition based on Andrea's original work. We dedicate this book to Andrea. She was passionate about improving maternity services. At Birth International, we pledge to continue Andrea's life's work.

Cover Illustration by Holly Priddis www.instagram.com/holly_reads_writes_creates/

Illustrations by Holly Priddis, Vesela Nenkova, Helen Brawley, Joanne Acty and Carol Lundeen

ISBN 978-1-922533-24-9

First Edition 1987
Second Edition 1994
Third Edition 1999
Fourth Edition 2003
Fifth Edition 2011
Sixth Edition 2021

Birth International
Sydney, Australia
Phone +61 2 9630 5357
Fax +61 2 8677 9532

Website: www.birthinternational.com
Email: info@birthinternational.com

Design and layout by Publish Central
Typeset by Midland Typesetters, Australia

One of the bestselling pregnancy books in Australia with over 500,000 copies sold

Disclaimer
While we've taken every possible care to provide accurate and up-to-date information on pregnancy, birth and parenting, this book isn't a substitute for midwifery or medical advice. If you are concerned about your own physical or mental well being or that of your baby, you should seek immediate assistance from a qualified healthcare provider.

Preparing
for Birth:

Mothers

Essential Information for Birth and Parenting

Jane Palmer and
Andrea Robertson

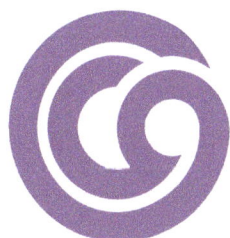

BIRTH
INTERNATIONAL

Contents

How to use this book

We've written this book as a simple, concise guide to pregnancy, birth and your new baby. The information supports what you'll learn in birth and parenting education courses. The book also serves as a reminder for the exercises that your childbirth educator will show you.

Check out our website if you want more information about the topics in this book or the references used. Our website is www.birthinternational.com.

The companion volume, *Preparing For Birth: Partners*, is a guide for fathers, partners and birth support people. Use the books together as a basis for making this pregnancy and birth uniquely yours.

When reading this book, you will find that it emphasises your involvement in birth and your active participation in labour. Many women want to be free to give birth using their ability and resources rather than being delivered of a baby.

You will only give birth to this baby once. Take your time to enjoy the discoveries of pregnancy and the richness that birth can bring to your life as a woman. We wish you the best for a healthy pregnancy, a happy birth experience and a wonderful time with your new baby.

Jane Palmer and Andrea Robertson

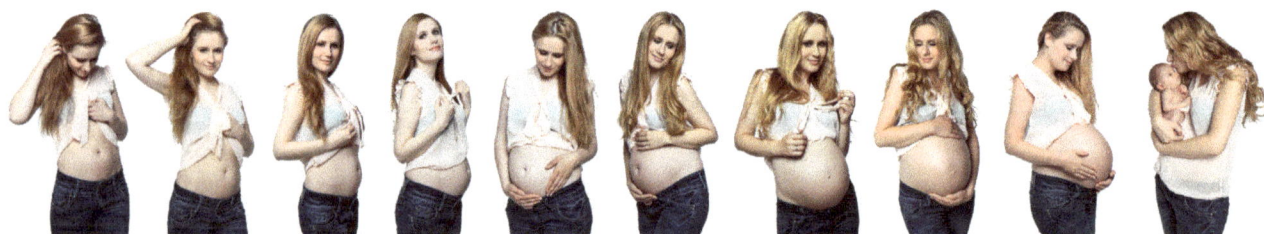

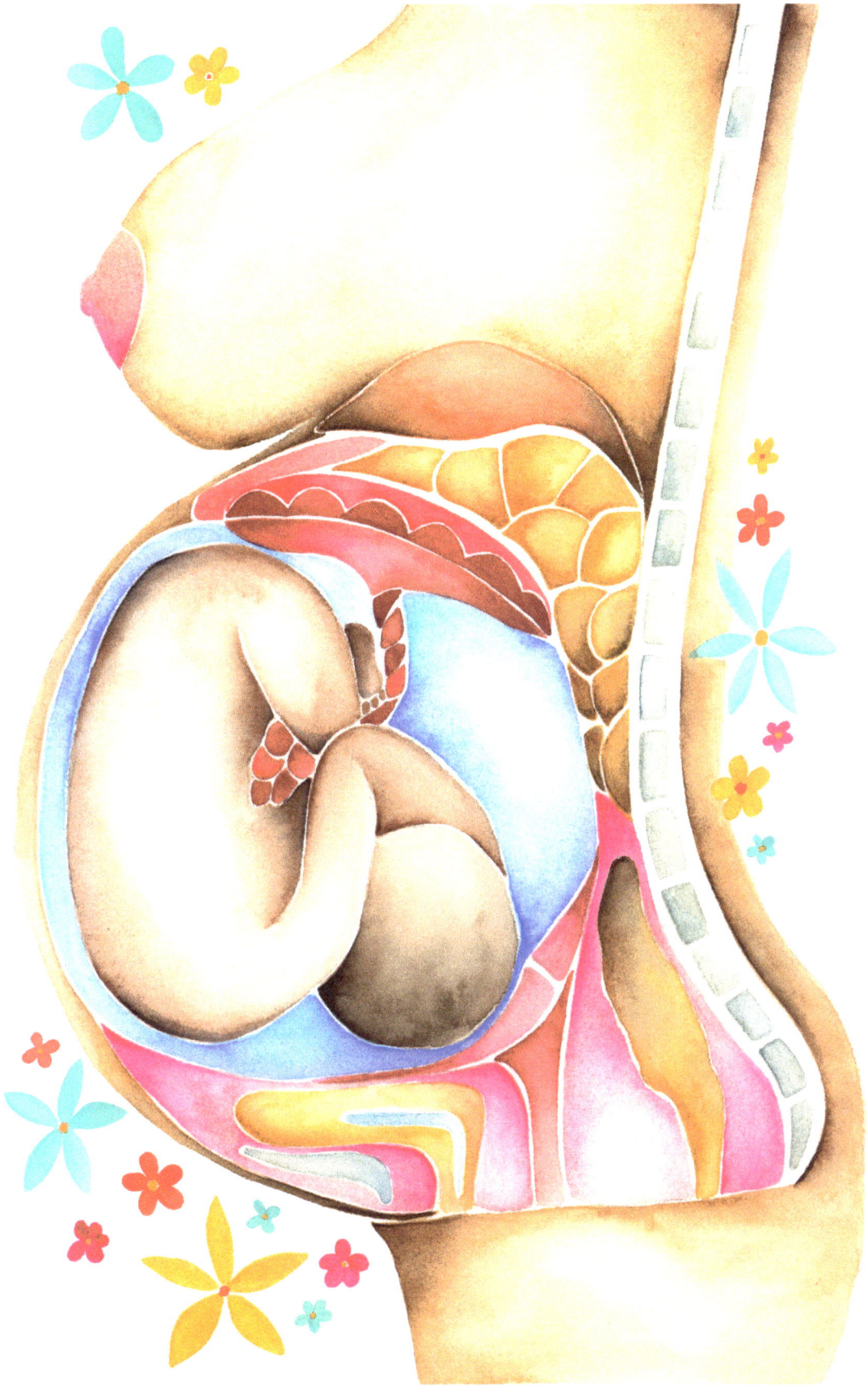

Your pregnancy

Eating wisely in pregnancy

Eating wisely in pregnancy and while breastfeeding means focusing on eating the most nutritious foods available. Nutrient-rich foods help you grow the healthiest baby possible. The popular view of eating for two suggests you need to eat a lot in pregnancy. The reality is that you only need to eat a little more to meet your needs, as well as your baby's. The quality of food is much more important than the quantity of food. Every woman's nutrient and energy needs are different.

> **You don't need to eat for two.**

Including quality snacks and eating smaller, more frequent meals will help reduce nausea and heartburn. Even better, it enables you to avoid feeling hungry and overeating. Avoid processed and ready-prepared foods, which are often high in salt, sugar and fats. Enjoy a wide variety of healthy foods each day.

Protein

Protein forms the building blocks of life. To build new cells, you need protein. Pregnant and breastfeeding women need around one gram of protein per kilo of body weight each day. If you don't eat meat, eggs or dairy products, you will need to get your protein from a balanced mix of other sources. Endeavour to eat a variety of protein-rich foods.

Primary sources of protein:

- red meat such as beef, lamb, pork, venison, kangaroo (preferably pasture-raised)
- poultry such as chicken, turkey, duck, quail (preferably pasture-raised)
- seafood and fish (preferably wild-caught)
- eggs (preferably from pasture-raised hens)
- cheese (preferably from pasture-raised animals)
- Greek yogurt (high in protein and low in carbohydrates)

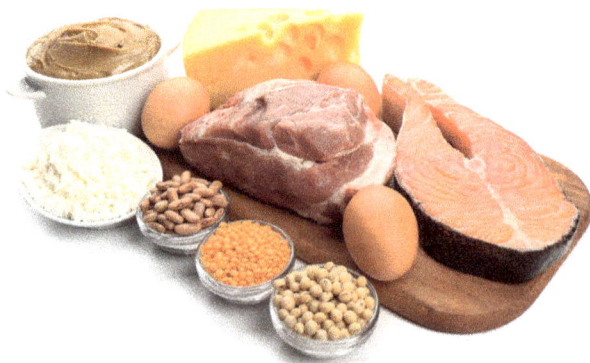

- nuts: almonds, brazil nuts, cashews, chestnut, hazelnuts, macadamias, pecans, walnuts and peanuts
- seeds: pumpkin seeds, sunflower seeds, chia seeds and quinoa
- nut butters: almond, peanut and cashew
- legumes: tofu, soybean, chickpea, mung bean and lentils

Vegetables

Vegetables are a powerhouse of vitamins and minerals. Low carbohydrate vegetables deserve a separate mention as ideally, they should make up around half of all the food you eat. Not only high in vitamins, they are also high in fibre and have little impact on blood sugar levels.

Lower carbohydrate and non-starchy vegetables are ideal and include:

- artichoke
- arugula
- asparagus
- beans
- beets
- bok choy
- broccoli
- Brussels sprouts
- cabbage
- carrot
- cauliflower
- celery
- cucumber
- eggplant
- garlic
- herbs (parsley, basil, rosemary, thyme, etc.)
- leeks
- lettuce
- mushrooms
- onions
- parsley
- peppers (green, red, yellow, etc.)
- radishes
- rhubarb
- shallots
- snow peas or pea pods
- spinach
- summer squash
- Swiss chard
- tomatoes
- turnips
- water chestnuts
- watercress
- zucchini.

Special nutrients in pregnancy

While all nutrients are essential in pregnancy, a select few play a unique role in maintaining a healthy pregnancy and supporting the growth and development of the baby.

- **Calcium:** Extra calcium is essential for healthy bone growth and strong teeth. Good calcium sources include dairy products, fish (especially with soft edible bones like canned pink salmon or sardines), leafy green vegetables, nuts, seeds, soy, tofu and calcium-fortified foods such as breakfast cereal.
- **Folate:** The need for folate increases substantially in pregnancy. Folate reduces the risk of neural tube defects in babies (an abnormality of the brain, spine or spinal cord). Foods rich in folate include green vegetables, legumes, rice, avocado, fruit and liver. The recommendation is to supplement with folic acid (a synthetic form of folate) for at least one month before pregnancy and the first 12 weeks of pregnancy.
- **Iodine**: Iodine is vital for your baby's brain development. Most women obtain a good portion of their iodine needs through a healthy diet and choosing iodised salt instead of the usual table salt. However, as many women have low levels of iodine in pregnancy, it's recommended that you take a supplement of 150 micrograms each day. If you have a thyroid problem, please seek advice from your midwife or doctor.
- **Iron:** In pregnancy, the body has an increased need for iron. Iron is essential for making red blood cells that carry oxygen around the body. Foods high in iron include red meat, chicken, fish, eggs, whole bread, cereal and green leafy vegetables. Some bread and cereals are iron-enriched. An iron supplement is only needed if you cannot get enough iron from your food and a blood test shows your iron levels are low.

Healthy menu ideas for pregnancy

Planning your meals while pregnant or breastfeeding can be tricky. A great way to work out what to eat is the plate method. It is much easier than worrying about portion sizes – you can visually see what you are eating on your plate. Aim for half your plate as non-starchy vegetables, a quarter of your plate carbohydrates and a quarter protein and fats.

For each main meal, use the following as a guide:

- two plus cups of non-starchy vegetables
- 85 to 110gms of protein foods
- ½ to 1 cup carbohydrate foods.

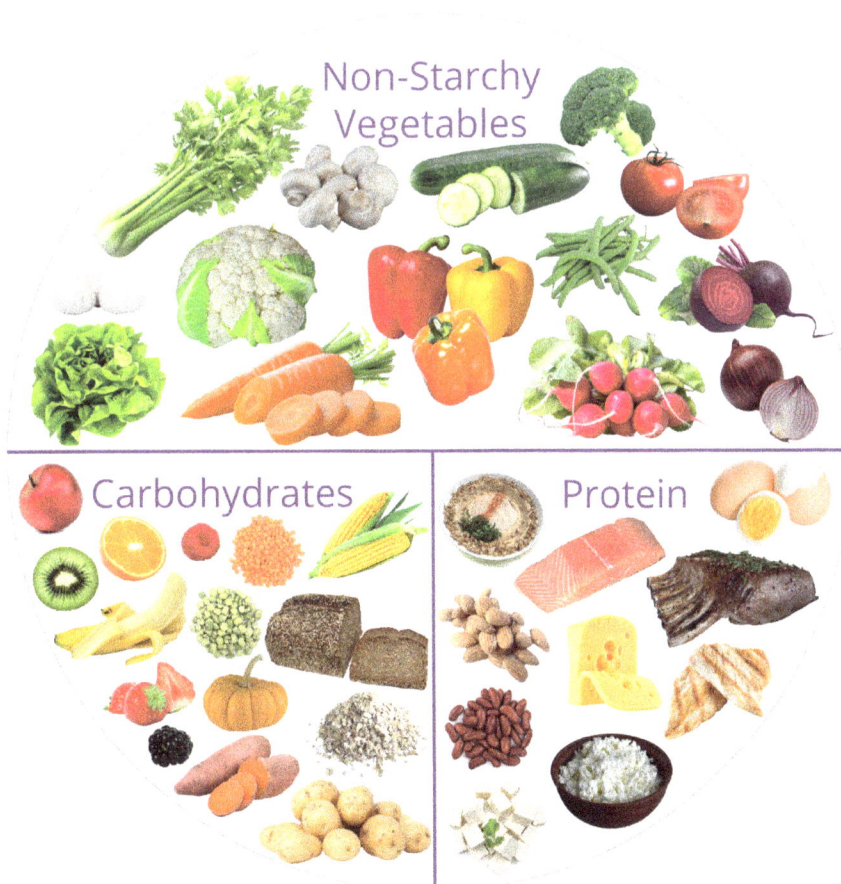

Non-Starchy Vegetables

Carbohydrates

Protein

Sample Menu	
Breakfast	• Cottage cheese, fresh fruit, pecans and cinnamon OR • Wholemeal toast, avocado and egg OR • Smoothie: Almond milk, banana, chia seeds, cinnamon and peanut butter
Morning snack	• Fruit with plain yogurt or a small amount of nuts OR • Wholemeal crackers, low-fat cheese and tomato
Lunch	• Grilled salmon, green salad, lentils, ½ avocado, olive oil and vinegar dressing OR • Coconut chicken curry, snow peas and corn on the cob
Afternoon snack	• Hommus with carrot sticks OR • Sardines in olive oil with celery
Dinner	• Marinated grass feed beef, roasted pumpkin, onion and zucchini OR • Slow-cooked pulled pork, green beans and roasted sweet potato chips

Foods to avoid in pregnancy

Some processed foods such as paté, soft cheeses (camembert, brie, blue-vein, ricotta), raw eggs, raw meat and poultry, ready-to-eat food and pre-cooked meals may contain listeria and salmonella bacteria. Either avoid these foods altogether or prepare and cook them thoroughly, as these bacteria can be harmful to your baby.

Avoid large predatory fish such as swordfish, marlin and shark, potentially containing high levels of mercury.

If you have allergies or are gluten or lactose intolerant, take care to avoid any foods that may cause you problems. Seek dietary advice to plan appropriate meals. You can reduce your baby's chances of developing allergies by planning to only breastfeed for at least the first six months.

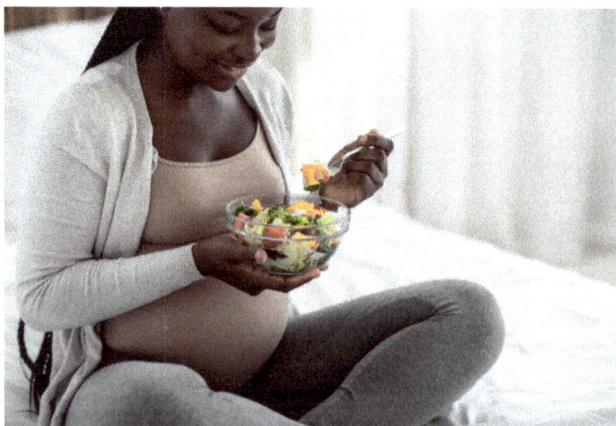

Avoidable hazards in pregnancy

Medications

Taking medication in pregnancy requires careful consideration. Medications include:

- prescription medications
- over the counter medicines
- pain relievers
- cough medicine
- antacids
- vitamin and mineral supplements.

There is the potential for the medication to cross the placenta and to affect your baby. While many preparations are safe, a small number can cause harm. Medications may have different effects at different stages of pregnancy.

Speak with your midwife or doctor about the benefits and risks of any medication you may need to take. This way you can make an informed choice. You may need to continue taking prescription medication for a medical condition. Or sometimes you can switch to a safer alternative.

Avoid exposure to chemicals around the house. Some substances are potentially damaging for your unborn baby. Chemicals include:

- insecticides
- cleaning agents
- garden sprays etc.

Ask your midwife or doctor if there is a local free *medication in pregnancy information service* to contact if you have any ongoing questions.

Alcohol

It's safest not to drink alcohol in pregnancy. Current research has not found a safe level of alcohol use in pregnancy. It's impossible to predict the effects on the unborn baby. Even small amounts of alcohol may be harmful to the baby's development. Babies most at risk are those whose mothers consume alcohol regularly or heavily on a 'binge'. However, the recommendation is that you avoid drinking any alcohol in pregnancy.

You may have drunk alcohol before you knew you were pregnant. The risk from drinking small amounts of alcohol in early pregnancy is low. Once you know you are pregnant, avoid alcohol. If you are concerned, speak to your midwife or doctor for information or support.

Smoking

Babies of mothers who smoke are at considerable risk of complications. Risks include being small-for-dates, born prematurely or stillborn. Babies whose mothers smoke also have a greater incidence of sudden infant death syndrome, chest infections and illness in their early years. The more a mother smokes, the greater the risks to her baby. We know that passive smoking (breathing in secondhand smoke) has a similar effect on the baby, although to a lesser degree than if the mother herself smokes. Shisha (waterpipe) smoking is harmful in pregnancy.

Caffeine

Due to its potential impact on the growing baby, the recommendation is to limit caffeine intake to 200mg per day. 200mg is approximately equal to either three cups of tea, two cups of instant coffee, four cola drinks or one expresso coffee per day.

As your baby grows

First trimester

The first three months of pregnancy are a significant period of change. You start to come to terms with the idea of being a mother and the physical changes occurring in your body.

Nausea or vomiting can be very distressing. Possible causes include changing hormone levels, fluctuations in blood sugar levels and blood pressure. A couple of dry crackers before rising in the morning, eating small meals often and avoiding smells that make you nauseous may help. Vitamin B6 can be beneficial and is in tuna, mackerel, bananas, sunflower seeds and hazelnuts. Ginger, in any form, can sometimes relieve nausea too.

Breast changes – at first, you may notice marked tenderness and tingling of the breasts, with sore nipples. Veins become prominent as the milk glands develop and the blood supply increases. Nipples also begin to darken.

Frequently passing urine is common in early pregnancy due to the pressure of your uterus on the bladder. Once the baby has grown up out of the pelvis, you should notice a significant improvement.

Vaginal discharge often increases. If it becomes excessive or smelly, it could be a sign of infection, and you should consult your midwife or doctor.

Tiredness and sleepiness are common in early pregnancy. Your body is adjusting to the physical changes involved in the rapid growth of the new body tissues.

By three months of pregnancy, your uterus rises above your pubic bone. You might be able to feel the fundus (top) of the uterus at this stage.

The baby lies inside the amniotic sac, floating in amniotic fluid. The image shows the placenta and cord.

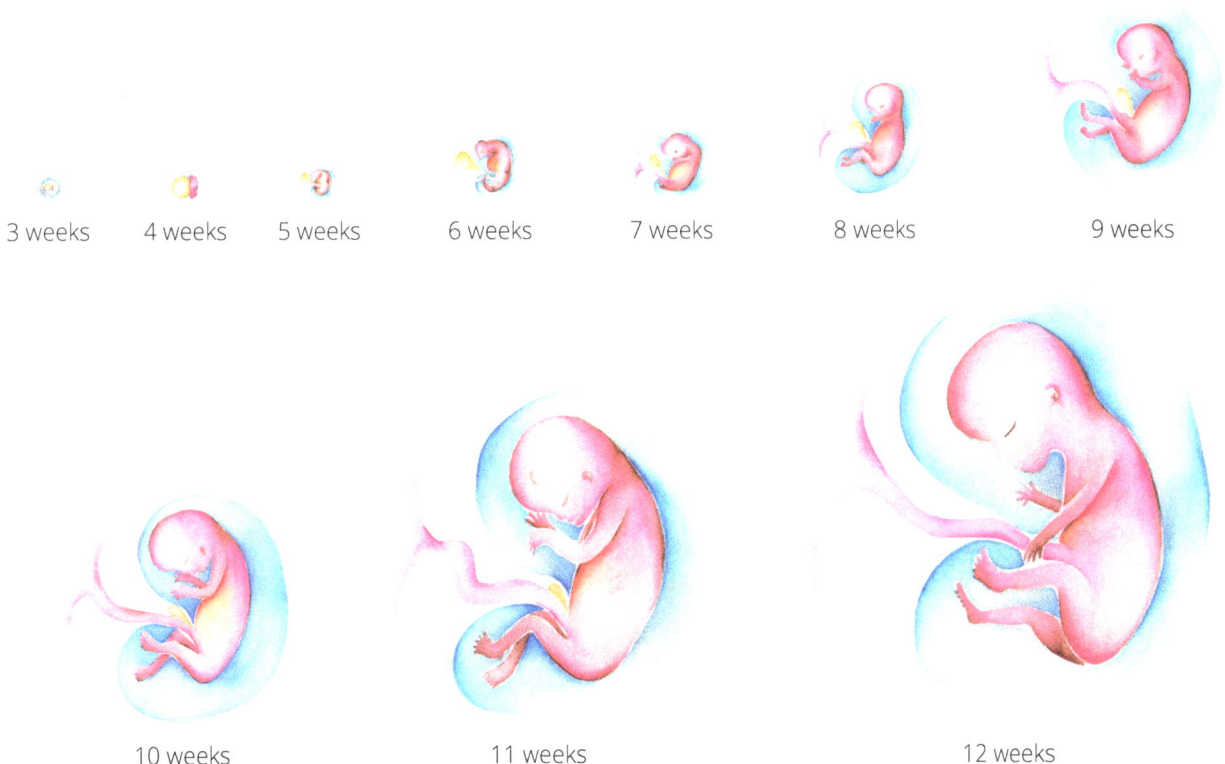

3 weeks   4 weeks   5 weeks   6 weeks   7 weeks   8 weeks   9 weeks

10 weeks   11 weeks   12 weeks

Second trimester

The second three months is usually the time of acceptance and planning. Women often feel fantastic physically, with the whole body working more efficiently. The placenta is now formed and operational, taking over the production of the pregnancy hormones. The uterus and baby are increasing rapidly in size.

Stretch marks may appear on your breasts, thighs and abdomen. Sometimes the skin feels dry and itchy, especially when there has been very rapid growth. Unfortunately, research shows oils and creams won't prevent stretch marks. They can, however, help keep your skin soft.

Colostrum is the earliest form of breast milk. Production starts from around 16 weeks. Some women notice colostrum leaking, and others don't. Leaking or not leaking colostrum has no relationship to the success of breastfeeding or milk supply. If necessary, you can wear a breast pad.

Heartburn, indigestion and constipation are all caused by the increased level of progesterone in the body. This hormone slows down the digestive system. Coupled with the pressure from the growing uterus, this causes these unpleasant side effects. Small frequent meals can help ease symptoms. Adding extra fibre and water to your diet will help constipation.

Urinary tract infections are common in pregnancy due to the action of progesterone on the urinary tract. Sometimes incomplete emptying of the bladder occurs. Contact your midwife or doctor promptly if you suspect a urinary tract infection.

Varicose veins may become noticeable in the legs, in the vulva or in the form of haemorrhoids. Varicose veins result from progesterone, causing increased softening of the blood vessel walls. Also responsible is the increasing pressure of the uterus on the pelvic veins. Resting with your legs up may help. Support stockings put on first thing in the morning can provide some relief.

Backache can be uncomfortable. One cause is the softening of the ligaments in the pelvis and lower back. Ideally, try to maintain a good posture with the bottom tucked in and shoulders back. Wearing flat-heeled shoes will help improve posture and avoid excessive pelvic tilting. Rocking the pelvis while on your hands and knees or resting leaning over a beanbag will ease the ache. See the exercise section for further ideas.

Your baby's movements usually start to be felt around 16–20 weeks. Sometimes these can be uncomfortable. You may also feel your baby having hiccups as well.

Third trimester

Braxton Hicks contractions usually become more noticeable in the last months of pregnancy. They are generally painless and come in bouts as the uterus goes through hardening and tightening periods. These contractions play a role in increasing circulation to the baby. Activity by either yourself or your baby can trigger them. As you approach your due date, they may increase in intensity and frequency. They can be mistaken for real labour contractions. Have a rest if you've been standing or walking. If they stop, you'll know they are Braxton Hicks contractions, not real labour contractions.

Breathlessness and heartburn become more common in the last months. Now the uterus is highest and pressing right against the diaphragm, ribs and stomach.

Engagement of the baby's head usually occurs in the last few weeks of the pregnancy as the pelvic floor muscles relax. The pelvic ligaments also soften in response to increased levels of pregnancy hormones. The heartburn and shortness of breath often improve as the baby's head descends into the pelvis. Once the head is well down, it is said to be 'engaged'. Engagement is a common sign that the body is getting ready for birth. But some babies don't engage until labour begins. However, this is more common with second or subsequent babies.

Urinary frequency is a common symptom of the baby's head engaging. The baby's head presses firmly on the bladder.

Cramps, muscle and nerve twinges, aching thighs and tired legs result from increased pressure within the pelvis. There is direct pressure on the nerves radiating out from the sacral area. Resting with legs elevated may help. Swimming is also beneficial.

Emotionally this is an exciting, uncertain time, as thoughts centre on the coming birth and being a parent. Increasing levels of endorphins may cause pregnancy amnesia. Endorphins can also make it hard to sleep, think straight and concentrate. Emotions can be changeable. Some women find themselves becoming more withdrawn and introspective, and others becoming more irritable.

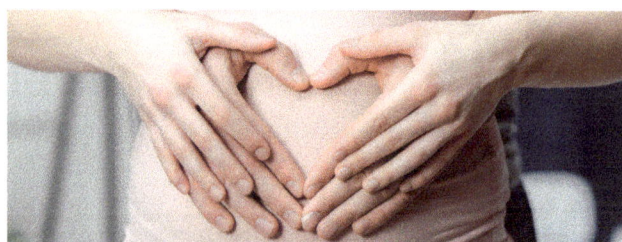

As the baby grows, the top of the uterus rises. In the last few weeks, the baby settles into the pelvis (engages), and the top of the uterus lowers slightly.

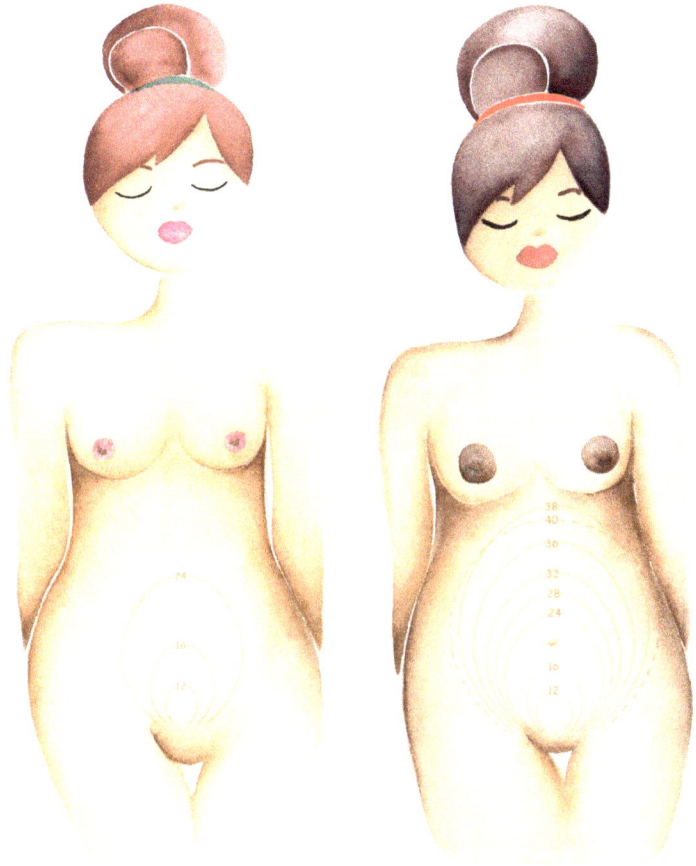

Weight gain in pregnancy

Gaining a healthy amount of weight in pregnancy is important to you and your baby's health. But how much weight should you put on? If you are in the healthy weight range, expect to gain around one to one and a half kilograms in the first 12 weeks, followed by one and a half to two kilograms per month until birth. If you are under or overweight, a healthy weight gain will vary. Check out the healthy weight gain in the pregnancy infogram below as a guide.

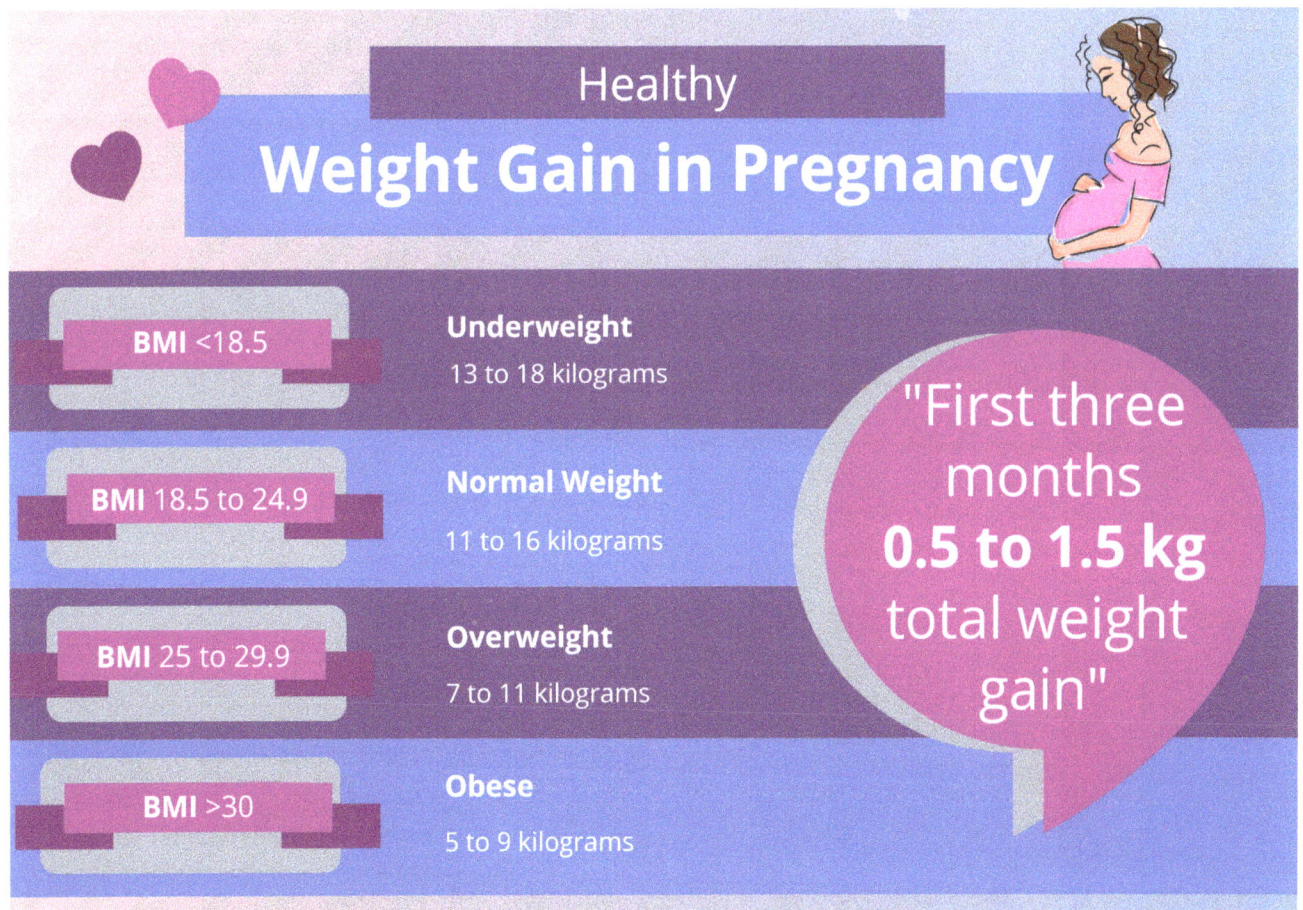

Healthy
Weight Gain in Pregnancy

BMI <18.5

Underweight
13 to 18 kilograms

BMI 18.5 to 24.9

Normal Weight
11 to 16 kilograms

BMI 25 to 29.9

Overweight
7 to 11 kilograms

BMI >30

Obese
5 to 9 kilograms

"First three months **0.5 to 1.5 kg** total weight gain"

Your due date

The consensus is that pregnancy lasts 40 weeks from the first day of your last menstrual period. For many women, however, this is not true. A term pregnancy is from 37 weeks to 42 weeks. But don't get excited thinking you'll more likely give birth before your due date. The average first-time pregnancy is around 40 weeks plus five days.

A subsequent baby's average arrival is a couple of days sooner than for a first baby. It's wise to accept that the magic 'estimated date of birth' is at best an approximation – the baby could arrive sometime before or sometime after that date. In the great majority of pregnancies, labour will begin when both mother and baby are ready. Your midwife or doctor may recommend an early ultrasound scan to estimate the baby's arrival date. Ultrasounds done before 14 weeks of pregnancy are accurate within a week on either side of your predicted date.

If there are concerns that your baby may be 'overdue' and you want to avoid an induction of labour, a couple of tests are available to determine the baby's health and wellbeing.

Sexuality

There may be completely unexpected changes in sexuality during pregnancy. It is hardly surprising that feelings of nausea and tiredness would reduce the desire for love-making, but apart from this, women do find that their sexual needs change. Some women find that their libido decreases significantly, while others find that this is when their desire increases more readily because of the increased tissue congestion in the pelvic region. Discussing these feelings with your partner will help them support your changing desires and help your relationship.

In later pregnancy, experimenting with different positions for sex may be necessary for comfort. Adapting positions can be a very positive time for sharing new ways of pleasuring each other.

If there has been a history of miscarriage with a previous pregnancy, your midwife or doctor may advise avoiding sex in the first three months of pregnancy. There are also some other conditions where having sex is not advisable. Talk to your midwife or doctor if you have any concerns.

However, it is safe in most pregnancies to have intercourse right up until birth, provided that it is comfortable and agreeable. Orgasm can cause strong contractions of the pregnant uterus, which some women find very uncomfortable, especially towards the end of pregnancy. Having sex will not cause spontaneous labour unless this was about to happen anyway. Some women do use sex to trigger labour if they are overdue and want to avoid an induction. Unfortunately, however, sex has not been found to bring on labour quicker.

Preparing for breastfeeding

Your body naturally prepares for breastfeeding during pregnancy. There is no need for you to do anything to prepare your nipples or breasts. The best way of avoiding problems is to learn as much about breastfeeding and normal newborn baby behaviour as possible during your pregnancy and have a list of support services on hand.

Many women find that as their breasts grow and become heavier, especially towards the end of the pregnancy, a well-fitting nursing bra provides comfort and support. Ideally, have these bras fitted by an expert.

Tips for breastfeeding success

The following suggestions for breastfeeding are worth considering while pregnant:

- Discuss your plan to breastfeed with your partner, family and support people, as well as your midwife or doctor.
- If you have a partner, get them on board. Research shows that supportive partners are important to breastfeeding success, particularly in the challenging early days.
- Learn about breastfeeding support services that you can get in contact with once the baby is born. Write down the contact details of:
  - the breastfeeding helpline ....
  - lactation consultant association ....
  - the early childhoood health nurse ....
  - local visiting midwives...
- Join the local breastfeeding association for woman-to-woman support.
- Attend a breastfeeding workshop. Hands-on preparation can provide you with a solid foundation of knowledge and skills for successful breastfeeding.

Expressing colostrum during pregnancy

Expressing colostrum (the earliest form of breast milk) may help if there's a possibility of separation from your baby following the birth. It can also be helpful if your baby needs extra breastmilk due to health issues with you (such as diabetes) or your baby. Limited research is available on expressing colostrum during pregnancy. If you are interested in expressing your colostrum, talk to your midwife or doctor before starting.

No breast or nipple preparation is required.

Exercise in pregnancy

General exercise

Exercise in pregnancy helps you stay healthy. Importantly physical activity throughout pregnancy is encouraged for all women who do not have medical restrictions. Exercise in pregnancy does not cause miscarriage, premature birth or problems with the baby.

Aim for at least 150 minutes of exercise per week of moderate-intensity, spread over three or more days a week. Walking is excellent and can be included in your daily routine. Swimming provides the perfect activity as the body becomes weightless in the water and offers vigorous exercise using all the main muscle groups. Stationary cycling and resistance training also are ideal in pregnancy.

If you have medical problems or pregnancy complications, check with your midwife or doctor before undertaking any exercise program.

Exercise will help strengthen muscles, increase circulation and support good posture. It also helps overcome fatigue and stiffness due to long periods of sitting (a common problem with some work). Even better, you can improve your health and that of your baby. Did you know women who are physically active throughout pregnancy have a lower risk of complications?

Women who've been very active before pregnancy can continue as long as they adjust their exercise program. Modify your usual exercise to match your capacity. It's essential to avoid high impact activities, exercising on your back, high-intensity balance work and excessive fatigue. Let your body guide you to a safe level of activity.

Remember to warm up and cool down, and drink extra fluids while you are exercising. Avoid overheating, as this can be harmful in pregnancy.

As your base heart rate is faster in pregnancy, it's challenging to monitor exercise by aiming for a target heart rate. It's easier and safer to use Borg's rating of perceived exertion (see the table below). During pregnancy, aim for moderate to hard intensity of exercise. Using the talk test, you can carry on a conversation while exercising without feeling exceedingly short of breath. Aim for level 3 to 5.

Talk Test Exercise Guide	
Borg Rating of Perceived Exertion	**Ability to Talk While Exercising**
0 Nothing at all	Easily carry on a conversation
1 Very Easy	Easily carry on a conversation
2 Easy	Easily carry on a conversation
3 Moderate	**Still able to carry on talking**
4 Somewhat Hard	**Still able to carry on talking**
5 Hard	**Still able to carry on talking**
6	Cannot talk continuously
7 Very Hard	Cannot talk continuously
8	Unable to talk at all
9 Extremely Hard	Unable to talk at all
10 Maximum Intensity	Unable to talk at all

RESEARCH SHOWS EXERCISE IN PREGNANCY CAN REDUCE RISK OF:

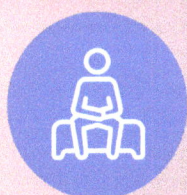 **67%** Depression

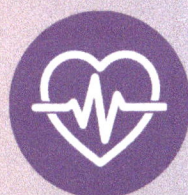 **40%** High Blood Pressure

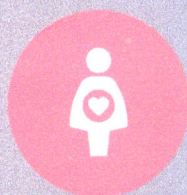 **38%** Gestational Diabetes

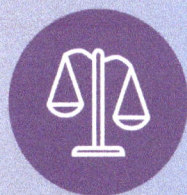 **32%** Excessive Weight Gain in Pregnancy

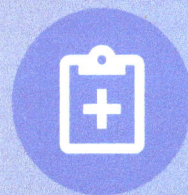 **15%** Caesarean Births

If you are doing yoga or attending group exercise classes, be sure to tell your instructor so they can adapt the exercises to accommodate your pregnancy.

Mix up your exercise to achieve more significant benefits. Recommendations are to do a variety of aerobic and resistance exercises. Also, research shows that adding yoga or stretching to your routine may be beneficial.

Finish each exercise session with some pelvic floor exercises, then give yourself a complete rest in a fully supported position as you consciously relax each part of your body. Arise and go out refreshed!

> **Keep cool while exercising – avoid overheating in pregnancy.**

Pelvic floor exercises

These exercises are essential for maintaining strong support for all your pelvic organs, especially your uterus and bladder. If you notice leakage of urine when you cough, laugh or sneeze, or are feeling a sense of heaviness in the vagina, this can be because of weak pelvic floor muscles. Please talk to your caregiver or see a specifically trained women's health physiotherapist.

Learn pelvic floor exercises now and practise them daily for the rest of your life! When you do these exercises, don't hold your breath or tighten your bottom, thighs or stomach muscles at the same time. Breath gently and relax.

Step 1

Sit forward on your chair and place your feet and knees wide apart. Place your elbows on your knees and lean forward. Your perineal area and vulva should be touching the seat now.

Step 2

Close your eyes, imagine that you want to stop yourself from passing urine or wind.

Step 3

Squeeze the muscles tightly around your back and front passages, lift your pelvic floor up and away from the chair. Count to eight and then relax for a few seconds. If you can't hold for eight, hold for as long as you can. Squeeze as tightly as you can, making sure you don't hold your breath. Try breathing out as you hold the squeeze.

Step 4

Repeat this squeeze and lift movement. Squeeze and lift several times until you notice the muscles tiring. At first, you may only be able to do this exercise three or four times in succession. With practice, you can aim to improve this number up to eight to 12 times.

Try to do a set of pelvic floor exercises several times each day. Once you've learnt how to do them correctly, you can do them anywhere.

Stretches

Helping your body become more flexible during pregnancy will make it easier for you to assume whatever positions you find comfortable during labour. You will also become more aware of how your body works and discover its limitations and capabilities.

Start the following exercises at any time in pregnancy; the earlier, the better. It is safe to exercise right up until you are due. Many exercises will help you overcome some of the discomforts of pregnancy, so even if you have only a few weeks before labour, you can benefit.

Do the exercises daily. You can combine them with other activities, such as watching television or reading. Even better, practise them with deep breathing (see page 25). If you have trouble with backache at work, 10 minutes of stretching exercises during your lunch break may ease your discomfort. Begin by holding each pose for as long as possible – even if only for a few seconds. Gradually increase this time until you can tolerate holding each pose for around two minutes.

> **Before doing any of the following stretches, consult a health professional specialising in pelvic pain in pregnancy if you have pelvic or lower back pain.**

Seated butterfly pose

Put the soles of your feet together. Place your back straight against a wall and your hands flat on the floor at your sides. Avoid bouncing the knees, which can cause injury through overstretching.

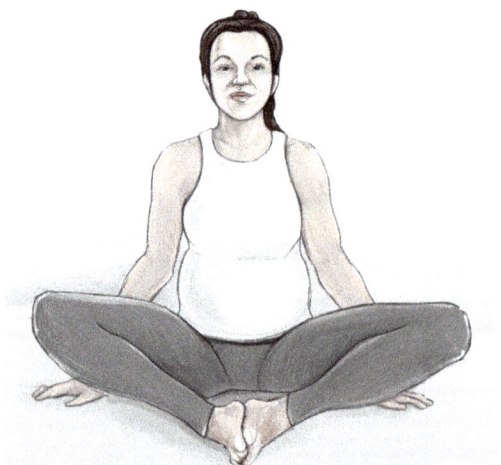

Sitting with legs apart

Sit on the floor with your bottom resting on the corner of a cushion. Spread legs apart with toes upwards. Using your hands at the sides, slide forward off the cushion to give an extra stretch. This exercise stretches muscles on your inner thighs.

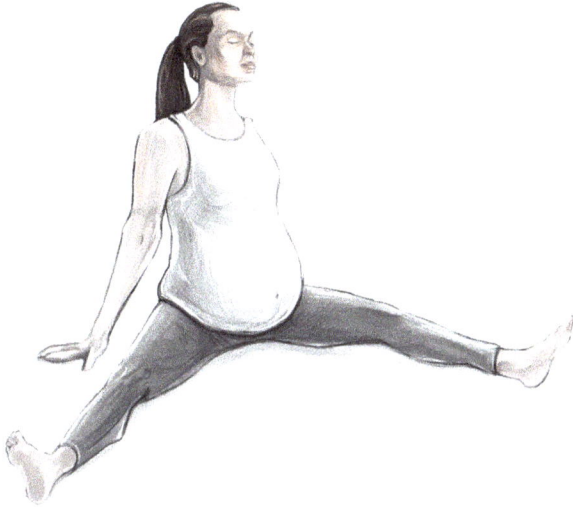

Squatting

Begin by squatting with heels raised and progress to having the feet flat. Pressing knees apart with the elbows will help with maintaining balance. Try these variations if you find unsupported squatting difficult.

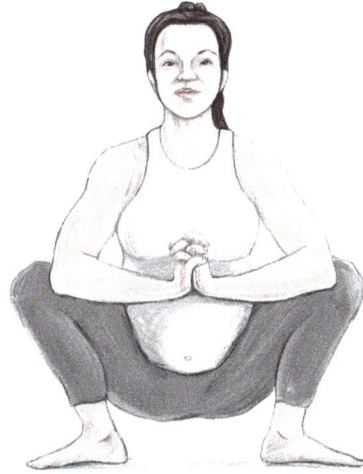

Calf stretches

Lean against the wall, with feet one in front of the other, toes pointing straight ahead. Bend your front knee, taking weight on the back leg. Repeat on the other side. This is a helpful exercise if you suffer from cramps in your legs.

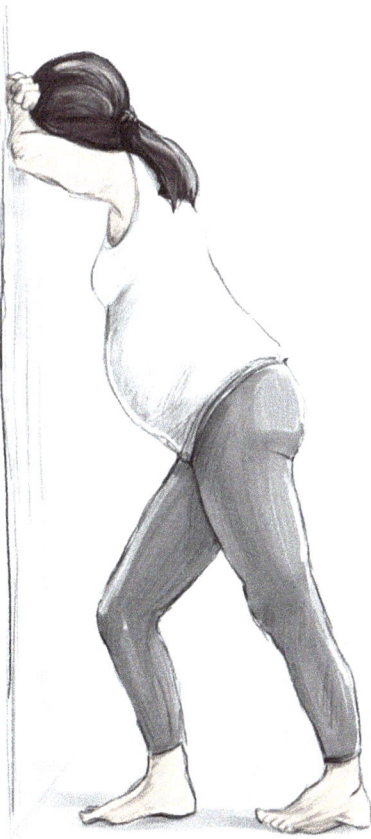

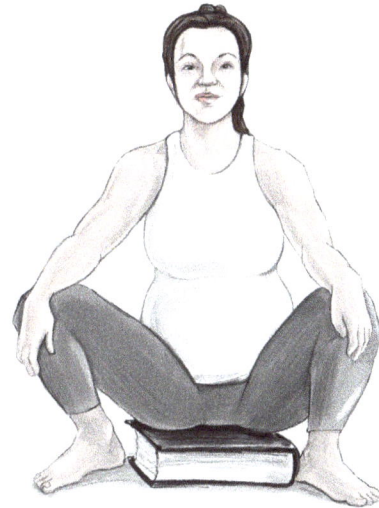

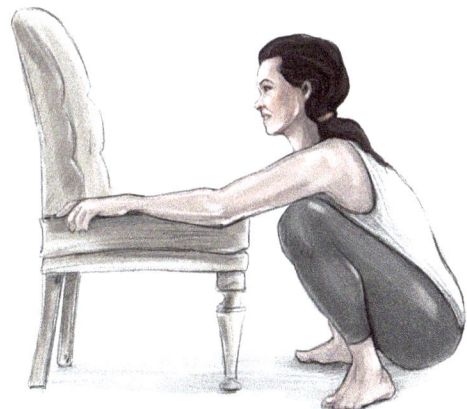

Exercises for easing back pain

Back pain is, unfortunately, commonplace in pregnancy. Exercise and stretching can help prevent or ease back pain. Here is a selection of stretches that are gentle and safe in pregnancy. If you have significant back pain, contact your midwife or doctor.

Forward stretch

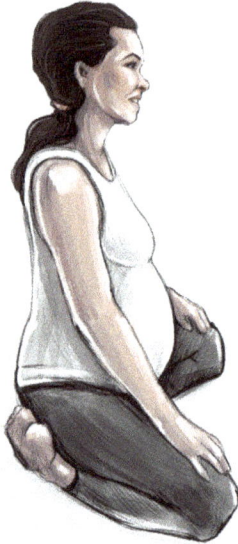

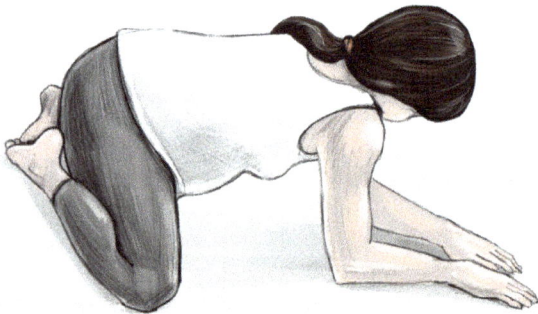

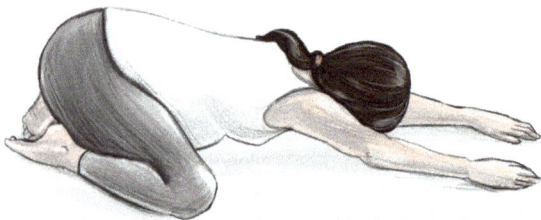

Begin by sitting on your feet, with toes pointed and touching. Bend forward from the hips, stretching your arms ahead and keeping your back straight. Slide forwards until you can place your elbows on the floor. Continue to extend your arms forward until your head can rest on the floor, keeping your back straight.

Cat-cow

This exercise series is excellent for easing backache and helping the baby into a good position for labour. Begin in a hands and knees position with your knees underneath your hips.

Cat

Round your back up, then straighten to level. Repeat several times at a moderate pace to rock your pelvis.

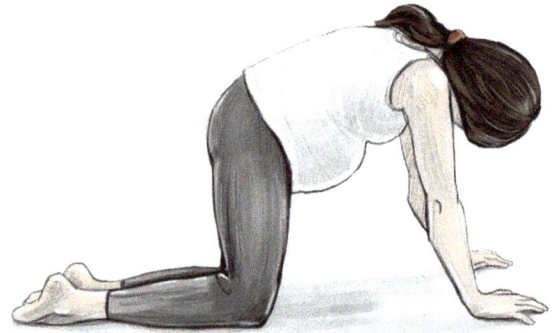

Cow

Gently arch your back, and let your belly go loose. Lift your head and tailbone towards the ceiling. Combine the cat-cow poses, flowing gently from one position to the other. Cat-cow warms your body and stretches your back and neck. Avoid going into an extreme cow position. If you have any discomfort, keep your back in a neutral position, without a bow in your back.

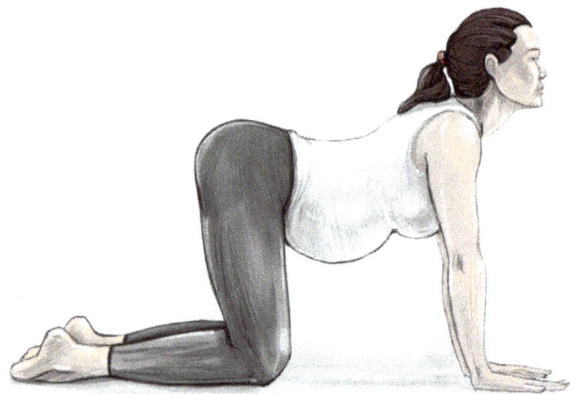

> **Exercise in pregnancy increases your chance of having a vaginal birth**

Middle back stretch

This stretch is an adaptation of the thread the needle yoga pose. A great stretch that opens the shoulders and stretches the spine. On hands and knees, tighten your abdominal muscles, extend one arm towards the ceiling, turn your head towards your raised hand.

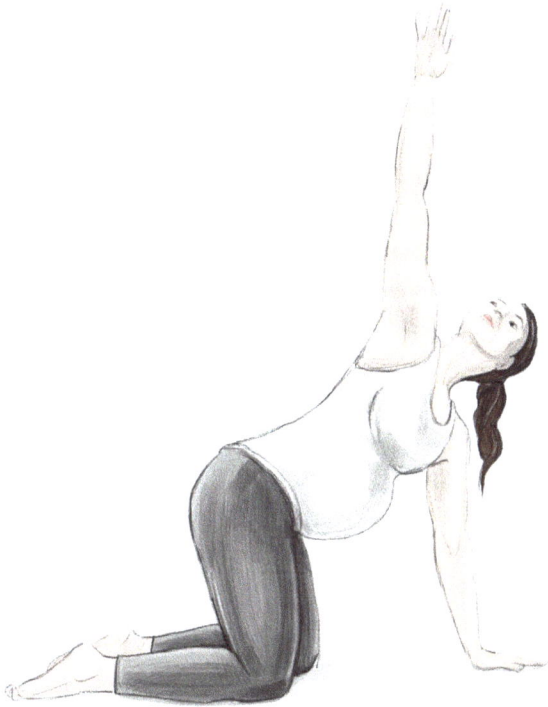

Then sweep your hand down and across your chest and behind your other arm. Reach across as far as you can. Your head follows your hand's movements.

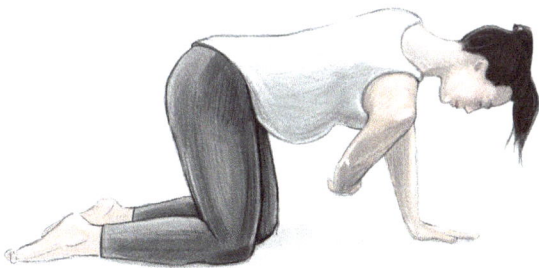

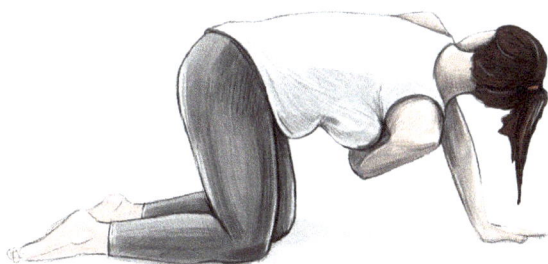

Pelvic rocking while standing

If you have back pain at work, you can ease it like this. Lean forward with your arms on a table or your desk and bend your knees slightly. You can rock your bottom gently back and forwards. Also, you can 'belly dance' by making circles with your hips. On your hands and knees is also a great position to do pelvic rocking.

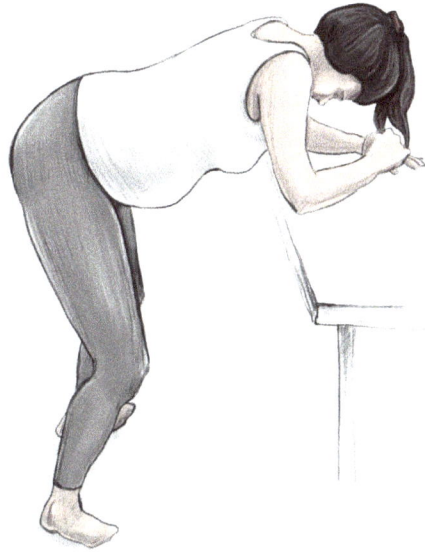

Healthcare in pregnancy

Throughout pregnancy, your midwife or doctor will check your health and the growth and development of your baby. They will plan with you a series of visits according to your needs. Healthy women need fewer check-ups than those with complications.

You will most likely be given a printed pregnancy record, which your caregiver updates at each visit. This record can is helpful if you need medical assistance when away from home. It also enables you to stay fully informed about the progress of your pregnancy.

Routine tests

The following are routine tests offered at each pregnancy visit:

- **Blood pressure** – Your blood pressure is normal if the top number is less than 140 and the bottom number is less than 90 (written 140/90).
- **Abdominal palpation** – feeling the baby's position and size.
- **Baby's heartbeat** – listened to after about 16 weeks.

- **Urine specimen** – not a routine test unless you have a clinical indication or other symptoms suggest a problem.
- **Your weight** – your midwife or doctor may offer you the opportunity to weigh yourself at each visit to identify low or high weight gain in pregnancy. Research is unclear if this is beneficial.

Tests for the mother's wellbeing

Your midwife or doctor will arrange for appropriate pregnancy tests, according to your history. Individual caregivers sometimes differ in the number and type of tests they order. Ensure you obtain copies of all test results, which will help you understand what is happening during your pregnancy.

Blood tests

Blood tests are ordered in early pregnancy to check:

- blood group and Rh factor
- haemoglobin level
- rubella antibody level
- exposure to infections such as syphilis, hepatitis B, hepatitis C and AIDS.

Later in pregnancy, blood tests may include:

- levels of glucose in the blood (24 – 28 weeks) to identify women at greater risk of developing gestational diabetes
- continuing levels of haemoglobin (28 weeks) to check for anaemia.

Other tests

Your midwife or doctor will offer you a urine test to look for a urinary tract infection that may not have any symptoms in early pregnancy.

Sometimes you'll be offered a vaginal swab around 35 to 37 weeks of pregnancy to identify potentially harmful bacteria that may infect the baby during birth. If present, the recommended treatment is antibiotics during labour.

If it's time for your cervical screening test, your midwife or doctor may offer it in pregnancy. Cervical screening in pregnancy is safe.

Tests to check the baby's health and development

All tests carried out during pregnancy, especially those to check on the baby's wellbeing, can be stressful for many women who find waiting for the results emotionally difficult. Screening tests are not diagnostic and are not foolproof, which means that false-positive and negative results can occur.

Before undertaking these tests, seek counselling and consider carefully, in advance, what you will do once the results are known.

Non-invasive prenatal test

Non-invasive prenatal testing (NIPT) is a relatively new test that's becoming increasingly available. Currently, guidelines don't exist as to who should have the test. Essentially the test involves taking the mother's blood from 10 weeks of pregnancy and looking at the baby's DNA in the blood for a few genetic abnormalities. NIPT is accurate in detecting Down syndrome and Edwards' syndrome. It's less accurate in detecting Patau's syndrome. NIPT can also identify the baby's sex and some sex chromosomal abnormalities.

NIPT is not a diagnostic test, meaning it can't diagnose a condition. The result provides a risk estimate.

On the upside, NIPT has a low false-positive result. For example, less than 1% of tests indicate that the baby may have Down syndrome when they don't. On the downside, it's a costly test and has a test failure rate of up to 4% (where they don't detect enough baby cells in the mother's blood). If the NIPT shows a high risk of abnormality, the usual recommendation is to have an amniocentesis or chorionic villus sampling.

Ultrasound

Ultrasound examinations use a hand-held scanner known as a transducer to transmit high-frequency sound waves to view what is happening inside the body. The sound waves reflect off different parts of the body back to the transducer, producing an image.

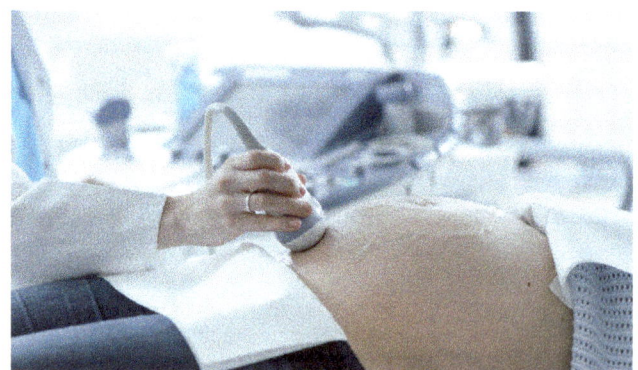

Since the late 1970s, the use of ultrasound in pregnancy is extensive. As with any medical procedure, there are benefits and risks. Although the general view is that ultrasound is safe in pregnancy, we don't know the long-term outcomes for babies, particularly those exposed to ultrasound multiple times. There are concerns about the potential biological effects on the body. Ultrasound can heat tissues – the significance of this is currently unknown.

Advantages of ultrasound include:

- excitement at seeing your baby for the first time and perhaps discovering your baby's sex
- provides an estimate of when your baby is due (and may help reduce the number of inductions of labour for babies suspected of being overdue)
- finding out if there is more than one baby
- detecting babies with a significant abnormality
- if there's bleeding in early pregnancy, ultrasound may predict whether a miscarriage will occur
- to follow up if there are any concerns with the pregnancy or baby.

Disadvantages of ultrasound include:

- research shows that routine ultrasound hasn't improved outcomes for mothers or babies
- overdiagnosis of problems, for example, errors in estimating baby's weight resulting in unnecessary intervention
- underdiagnosis of issues, for example, missing approximately 50% of abnormalities
- lack of high-quality scientific studies looking at the effect of modern high-powered ultrasound machines on babies.

Using ultrasound for non-medical reasons to gain a keepsake is discouraged.

The first trimester

Dating ultrasound confirms the position and number of babies and calculates the baby's approximate due date. The gestation for this ultrasound is between 6 and 12 weeks.

The second trimester

Nuchal translucency is a screening test that provides a statistical estimate of risk. The ultrasound looks at lots of things, including the thickness behind the baby's neck. A sample of the mother's blood is also taken. Information from these two tests, along with your age, weight and your baby's gestational age, is entered into a computer, and it produces a risk score for conditions such as Down syndrome. The ideal gestation for this screening is between 11 and 13 weeks.

Morphology ultrasound is done at 18 to 20 weeks and is a detailed ultrasound examination to identify abnormalities in the baby, placenta, umbilical cord, fluid around the baby and your cervix. The baby's sex can also be determined if requested by the parents.

Third trimester

Your midwife or doctor may recommend a *fetal welfare ultrasound* if your pregnancy is high risk or to check on the location of a low-lying placenta.

Chorionic Villus Sampling (CVS)

A CVS is a test for fetal abnormality sometimes offered to women in high-risk groups, usually between 11 and 14 weeks of pregnancy. A small sample of tissue from the placenta (the chorion) is removed under ultrasound guidance and tested to exclude abnormalities such as Down syndrome, inherited disorders and sex-linked diseases such as muscular dystrophy and haemophilia.

CVS has a greater than 1% chance of miscarriage, and in up to 3% of women, CVS will be unsuccessful, resulting in the need to repeat the test.

Results of a CVS are usually available within two to three weeks. Early diagnosis enables parents to decide whether or not to continue the pregnancy. Termination, if desired, is easier in the first trimester.

Amniocentesis

During an amniocentesis, a doctor uses ultrasound to guide a long needle through the mother's abdominal wall and into the amniotic sac. Ultrasound helps ensure that the baby and the placenta are out of the way. Using a syringe, the doctor withdraws a sample of amniotic fluid.

The baby's cells are collected from the amniotic fluid and grown in a laboratory. A scientist then examines the cells for genetic abnormalities. Abnormalities include Down syndrome and structural problems such as spina bifida. Usually performed at 15 to 18 weeks of pregnancy, the results take 10 to 21 days to arrive. Therefore if parents choose a termination based on the amniocentesis result, the pregnancy will be advanced.

The risk of miscarriage is around 1%.

Cardiotocograph (CTG)

A midwife or doctor may recommend a CTG in pregnancy if you're overdue or concerns exist about your baby's wellbeing. A CTG machine records the baby's heartbeat and any contractions of the uterus onto paper. A midwife or doctor interprets the resulting paper trace. A suspected unwell baby may result in the recommendation of induction of labour or even a caesarean birth. See pages 54 and 55 for further information on CTG.

Keeping your baby safe

Monitoring baby's movements

Monitoring your baby's movements is an easy way to keep track of your baby's health. Every baby moves differently, so getting to know your baby's movement pattern is important. No ideal number of movements exist. Take note of the strength, frequency and pattern of your baby's movements.

Getting to know your baby's movements gives you the confidence to let your midwife or doctor know if you notice changes in the movement pattern. Around 55% of women who experienced stillbirth noticed that their baby's movements slowed beforehand.

You will start to feel your baby move somewhere between 16 and 24 weeks of pregnancy. First movements are usually soft but gradually become stronger. From approximately 24 weeks of pregnancy, most babies settle into a pattern of movements.

Trust your instincts. Don't delay seeking help if you are concerned about the reduced movements of your baby. Phoning a midwife or doctor is essential. Help is available 24 hours a day, 7 days a week.

> **Babies don't move less towards the end of pregnancy.**

Safe sleeping

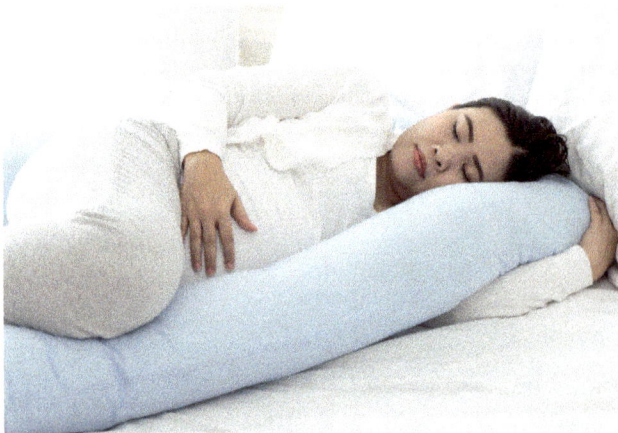

Women report concerns about sleeping. After 28 weeks of pregnancy, the recommendation is to sleep on either the left or right side. If you sleep on your back, this causes a reduced blood supply to the baby. By side sleeping, you reduce the chance of stillbirth by half.

While you sleep, you will change your position. If you wake up on your back, don't worry; switch your position back to side-lying. The most important thing is going to sleep on your side, not the position you wake up.

As the uterus grows more prominent and the baby becomes more active, it is often increasingly difficult to sleep. The need to empty your bladder through the night adds to sleep becoming broken and restless.

Towards the end of the pregnancy, the endorphin levels (the body's natural opiate) rise further, making sleep elusive. Dreams increase in frequency, too. To help with sleep, try repositioning your body using extra pillows to take the weight of your legs off the uterus.

Raising your head and shoulders with extra pillows will help avoid heartburn and indigestion. Chamomile tea before bed may also help. Relaxation exercises, a back rub or stretching before bed may also help relieve tension and make sleep easier.

If you suffer from cramps, try using a pillow at the end of your feet to keep the bedclothes' weight off your legs. Positioning the pillow this way will help you avoid pointing your toes, which frequently triggers severe muscle cramps.

> **Sleep on your side from 28 weeks of pregnancy. Either side is fine.**

Every week counts

The timing of birth is a huge issue. With increasing intervention rates, such as the early induction of labour and caesarean birth, the number of babies born before 40 weeks will increase. Most babies will be born between 37 to 42 weeks, so why is a birth before 39 to 40 weeks an issue? A baby still has more growing to do, particularly brain development. In the last five weeks of pregnancy, a tremendous amount of growth is occurring. It's best, where possible, to allow a baby to choose their birthday (let labour start naturally).

What are the differences for your baby if born at different gestations (weeks of pregnancy)? In a nutshell, the earlier the baby is born, the higher the risk of needing admission to a neonatal nursery. The earlier a baby is born, the more likely they are to have difficulties at school. To give babies the best chance, and reduce the risk of separation from their parents, talk about the timing of birth with your midwife or doctor.

To understand the complete picture, visit www.everyweek counts.com.au

Don't worry if your labour starts naturally at 38 to 39 weeks; your baby is signalling they are ready to be born.

Every week of pregnancy counts

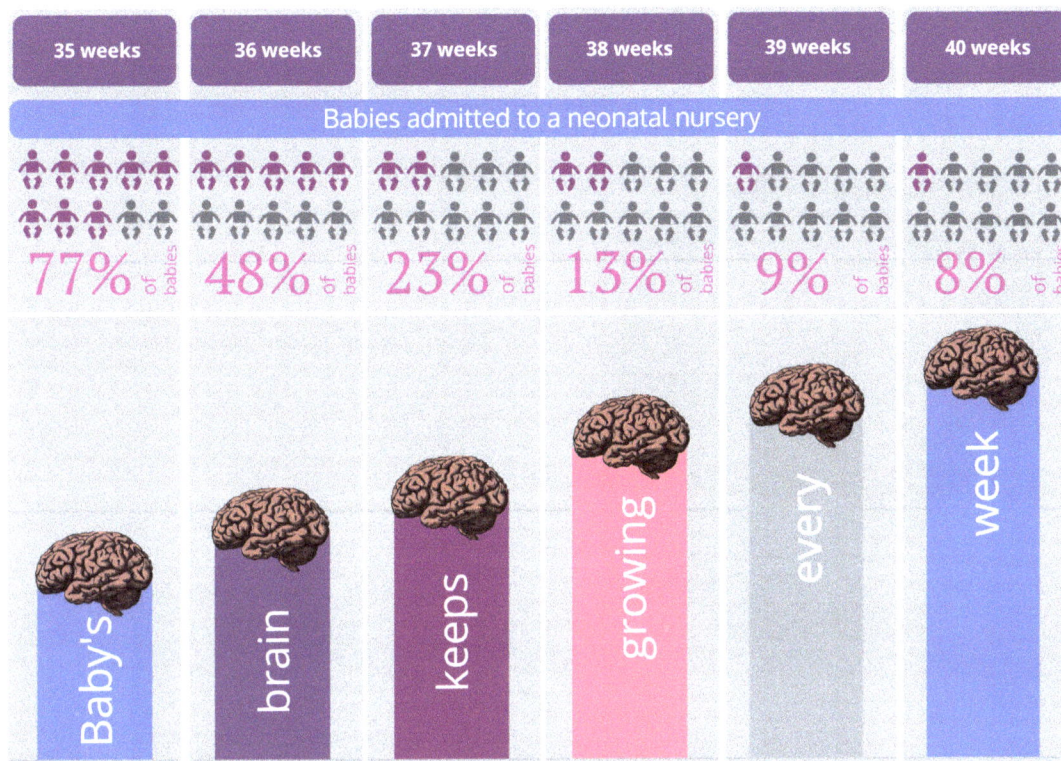

35 weeks	36 weeks	37 weeks	38 weeks	39 weeks	40 weeks

Babies admitted to a neonatal nursery

77% of babies	48% of babies	23% of babies	13% of babies	9% of babies	8% of babies

Baby's brain keeps growing every week

Increased risk of having difficulties at school

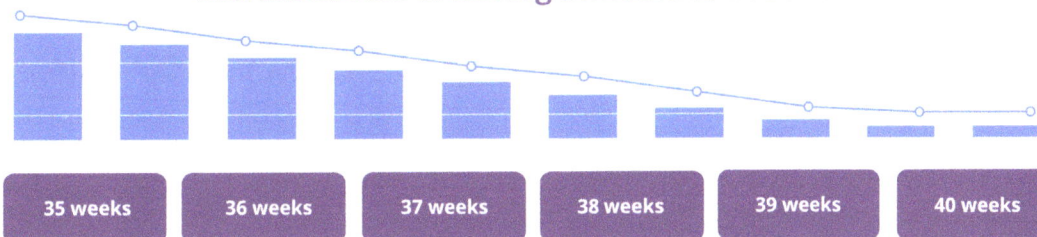

35 weeks	36 weeks	37 weeks	38 weeks	39 weeks	40 weeks

Mind-body connection

Understanding the mind-body connection gives a better insight into labour and birth. Negative emotions such as fear or stress cause the release of hormones that stop or slow contractions. Positive emotions such as confidence and feelings of safety increase the release of the hormone oxytocin, making contractions of the uterus happen. In a nutshell, your thoughts and emotions have the potential to affect the course of labour and birth. The mind-body connection is powerful.

You can do many things to improve the mind-body connection:

- eat well
- exercise
- take a warm bath
- talk about your fears

- learn more about your body, labour and birth
- practise relaxation and deep breathing
- enjoy massage.

We'll explore some of these aspects to improve the mind-body connection in the coming sections.

Hormones of birth

When you are giving birth, a complex system of hormones is working together in your body. In this section, we'll explore how your brain and hormones affect labour. Also, we'll look at what increases and what decreases oxytocin, so you'll know what makes labour go more smoothly.

Oxytocin

Oxytocin is known as the 'hormone of love'. Oxytocin flow stimulates labour contractions. The higher levels of natural oxytocin mean more frequent and efficient contractions, making labour shorter. A deep part of our brain controls the release of oxytocin. For this part of the brain to work effectively, set the environment so you can let go of your thoughts and follow your instincts.

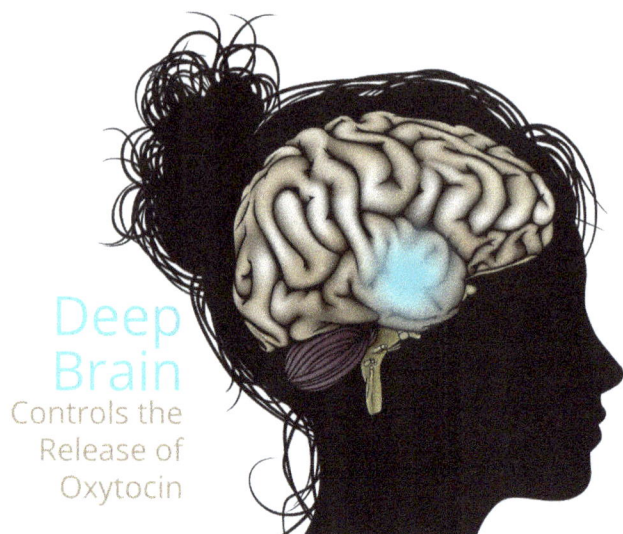

Deep Brain
Controls the Release of Oxytocin

Endorphins

Endorphins are known as happy hormones. Everyone produces endorphins and at individual levels. Levels rise throughout pregnancy and peak towards the end of labour. Endorphins have pain-relieving qualities, so they help reduce the pain you feel. They also create an amnesic effect, making you forgetful and vague. With a feel-good factor, they help you feel euphoric after birth.

Adrenaline

Everyone produces adrenaline when faced with danger. The release of adrenaline is an instinctive, involuntary reaction to a threat. It's a natural safety mechanism over which we have no conscious control. Sometimes known as the stress hormone, adrenaline is responsible for the fight-or-flight response.

The fight-or-flight response can cause us to feel our heart rate increase, a dry mouth, agitated, and cold and clammy. Another effect is that adrenaline redirects blood flow to major muscles to fight the threat or run away. While doing this, it diverts blood away from non-vital parts of the body, including the uterus. Reduced blood flow to the uterus, over time, increases the risk of the baby becoming distressed. When a woman feels unsafe, labour will slow or stop altogether as instinctually, her body inhibits the labour without conscious control.

When you don't feel comfortable, you start to use the thinking part of your brain. This front part of the brain is called the neocortex. In labour, you want to switch off the thinking part

of your brain, so your body uses the deep part to help you labour and give birth.

Release of excessive adrenaline results in:

- reduced oxytocin –> slowing labour
- reduced endorphins –> more pain
- altered contractions of the uterus –> dilatation of the cervix (opening of the uterus) slows or stops
- reduced blood supply to uterus and baby –> baby becoming distressed.

The effects of adrenaline are quickly reversed by:

- removing the source of fear
- creating an emotionally safe environment
- reducing sensory stimulation (like turning down the lights, stopping any noise, warming the room, and removing unnecessary people)
- using water in labour (see page 40)
- having a supportive team
- understanding what is happening.

Melatonin

Your brain produces melatonin in response to darkness. Created by the pineal gland (also located in the deep brain), melatonin causes relaxation and, notably in labour, works alongside oxytocin to enhance contractions. Melatonin peaks at night, which may be why many labours start at night.

Prolactin

Prolactin is known as the mothering hormone. It's a primary hormone involved in breastfeeding. In pregnancy, levels start to increase and prolactin peaks when you give birth. It's thought prolactin works alongside oxytocin to enhance labour.

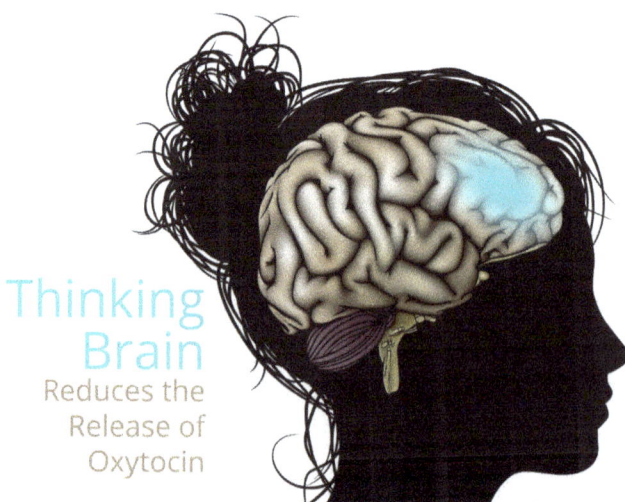

Thinking Brain
Reduces the Release of Oxytocin

Hormones of birth

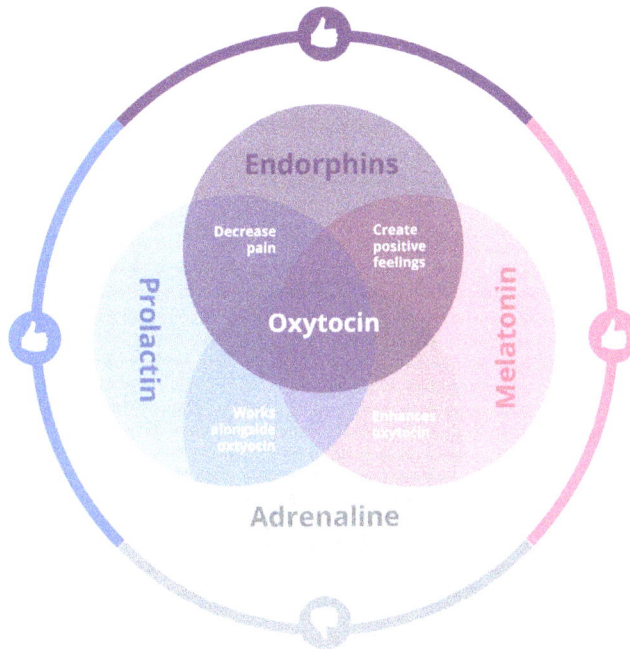

Endorphins
- Decrease pain
- Create positive feelings

Oxytocin

Prolactin — Works alongside oxytocin

Melatonin — Enhances oxytocin

Adrenaline

Fear-tension-pain cycle

The fear-tension-pain cycle is a concept developed by Dr Grantly Dick-Read. In simple terms, the more fearful a person is, the more tension they feel, the more pain they experience and the more fearful they become. In this cycle, increasing adrenaline levels slow labour and make it more painful.

When you are in labour, you want to aim for the opposite of the fear-pain-tension cycle. The aim is to increase hormones that enhance labour and decrease adrenaline. Aspire to the positive birth cycle. We'll explore all aspects of the positive birth cycle in the coming sections.

FOR A SAFE AND EFFECTIVE LABOUR
High oxytocin levels >> Efficiency
High levels of endorphin >> Comfort
Low levels of adrenaline >> Faster labour

Breaking the Fear-Tension-Pain Cycle

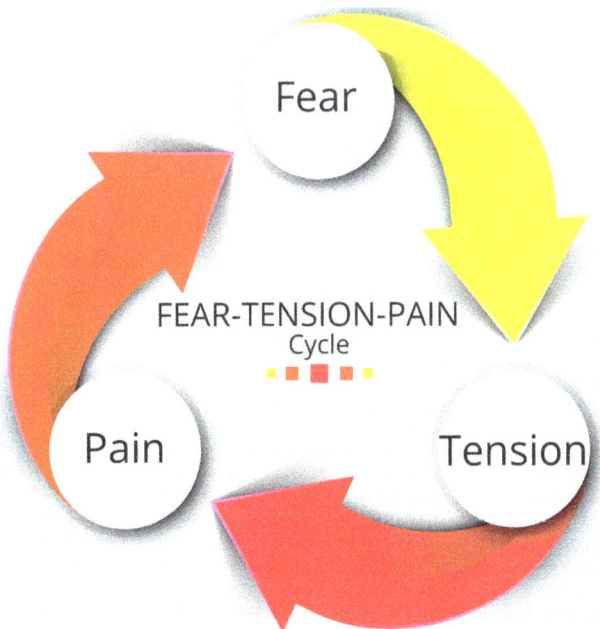

FEAR-TENSION-PAIN Cycle
- Fear
- Tension
- Pain

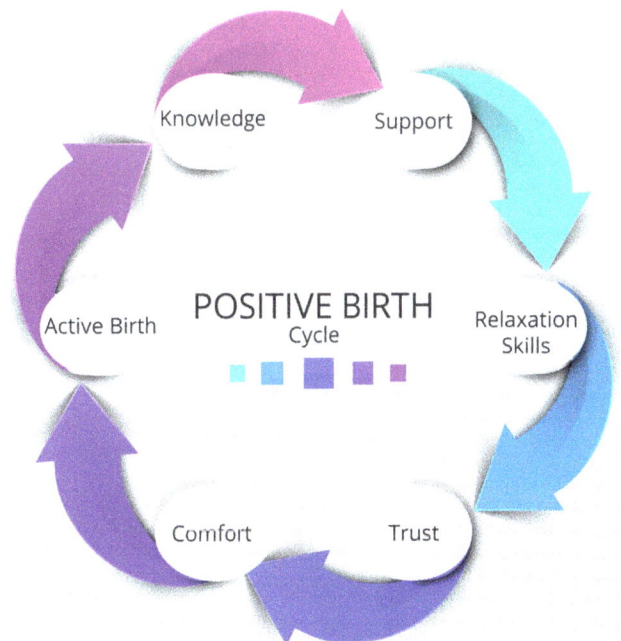

POSITIVE BIRTH Cycle
- Knowledge
- Support
- Relaxation Skills
- Trust
- Comfort
- Active Birth

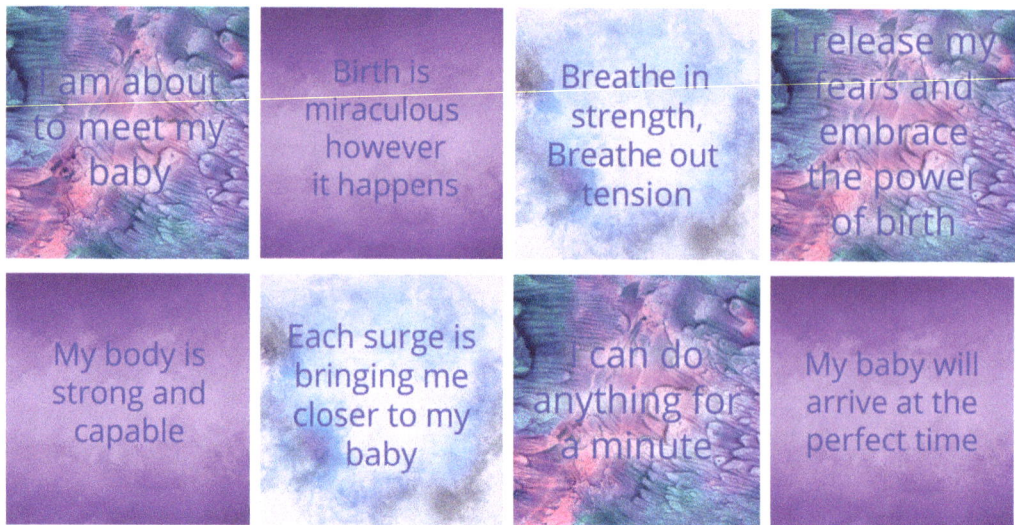

I am about to meet my baby

Birth is miraculous however it happens

Breathe in strength, Breathe out tension

I release my fears and embrace the power of birth

My body is strong and capable

Each surge is bringing me closer to my baby

I can do anything for a minute

My baby will arrive at the perfect time

Positive self-talk

Research shows that positive self-talk changes the way your brain processes information. A great way to feel confident about giving birth to your baby is by writing down or reading positive affirmations. Positive affirmations are positive statements about labour, giving birth and meeting your baby. These statements are personal and meaningful to you. Examples of positive affirmations include those shown in the image above.

Are you stuck on ideas? There are plenty of positive affirmations online. You can print them or create them artistically to put on your wall. You can even record your positive affirmations to background music and listen to a recording. Alternatively, download an MP3 of positive birth affirmations – there are free and paid versions available.

Use this section to write down your positive statements for birth:

....

....

....

....

Listening to an affirmation recording while you are in labour can be encouraging.

Reducing fear

It is common for women to experience fear before giving birth, particularly if this is their first baby. For 6 to 10% of women, this fear is overwhelming and they need professional support. For others, acknowledging fear, doing what is possible to reduce the fear and understanding that it may not be possible to eliminate it totally is invaluable.

Talk about your fears

Talk it out with your partner, midwife, doctor, friend, doula, social worker or psychologist. Finding the right person to explore your fears with and help put things into perspective is invaluable. If possible, avoid scary stories. Women often share stories of their traumatic births. If you find these stories are making you anxious, ask women not to share their birth stories.

If you can't find the right person, ask your midwife or doctor for a referral to a psychologist or social worker with a particular interest in pregnancy and birth. Attending a few sessions with a mental health professional can be amazingly effective.

Gather your tools

Knowledge can help reduce fear. Attend birth and parenting education classes. Put a plan in place for which tools you will use for labour; for example, active birth positions, massage, water, relaxation strategies, non-pharmacological and pharmacological ways of increasing comfort in labour. For some women, creating a list of birth preferences is helpful (see page 30).

Look after yourself, your mind and your body. Exercise as much as you can and practise relaxation (see page 25). Research shows that practising meditation may help ease fears of birth. You could consider downloading a meditation app for your phone (there are ones specifically designed for pregnant women).

Find the right support

Gather your support team around you. Choose people who are on the same page as you are. Make sure they are encouraging, calming, reassuring and not discouraging. Most importantly, you need to feel comfortable being able to let go in front of them without judgement. Also, consider continuity of care from a known midwife. Many hospitals now offer caseload midwifery care (see *Preparing for Birth: Partners* for choosing the best maternity care).

> **When you are in labour, if fear occurs, deal with it as best you can by doing what feels right. Fear will pass, labour will continue and you will give birth.**

Relaxation

Pregnancy, birth and the early days after birth can be stressful for new parents. It is worthwhile to learn ways of reducing this stress and some specific techniques to relieve its symptoms. You can practise these techniques with your partner at any time in the pregnancy, and you may also find them helpful after the baby is born.

General relaxation

Find a comfortable position where your body is fully supported, perhaps by sitting and leaning forward over some cushions with your head resting on your folded arms or propping yourself up in a comfortable chair with a pillow behind your head. Pay attention to your legs and feet – they should be relaxed and comfortable. Playing soothing music will help you tune out any nearby distractions.

Take several slow, deep breaths, releasing any tension from your body each time you breathe out. Working from your feet up through your body, imagine each part is getting heavier, looser, sinking into the chair seat or pillows. Continue until you have achieved a state of overall relaxation, allowing yourself time to enjoy the sensation of complete release for several minutes before gradually re-energising through first wriggling your feet, then legs and arms.

You can do this progressive muscle relaxation anywhere provided you can rest your head, and your body is well supported. It can also be helpful if you are having trouble falling asleep.

Visualisation

Visualisation is a relaxation technique using guided imagery, usually either as a recording or with someone speaking directly to you. Generally, music accompanies the script to enhance the relaxation effect. Using this technique, you focus on the spoken word to help you relax and encourage positive thoughts on pregnancy, birth or parenting. While not for everyone, if you find your mind wanders off during general relaxation, this might be a preferable relaxation option. You can record a guided visualisation script yourself. Alternatively, try searching online for 'guided visualisation for birth' or 'guided imagery for birth'.

Breathing

You can use breathing techniques to slow things down and engage the primitive part of your brain that releases birth hormones. Use your breath to release tension in labour and help maintain a relaxed state. The rate at which you breathe is an individual one, but try to breathe as slowly as you can at all times. There is no need to learn how to breathe in labour – you already know how to do this, and your body will automatically adjust the rate as needed. As the body requires more oxygen and energy, so you will breathe a little faster.

Patterned breathing or breathing to certain 'levels' within the chest can create tension and is very tiring. This kind of distraction technique often fails to work when more intense contractions develop towards the end of the first stage. By using relaxed, deep breathing at your own pace, you will find you can conserve energy and stay calm, in tune with the rhythms of your labouring body.

Abdominal breathing is a technique with extensive positive research. Sometimes called diaphragmatic breathing, this technique is where your stomach goes in and out as you breathe. Abdominal breathing is slow, controlled breathing often used with yoga or meditation. Benefits include decreasing adrenaline, increasing the relaxation response and lowering blood pressure.

Music

Research shows music may help decrease pain in labour and help women feel more satisfied with labour. But what type of music? Music choice is very individual. Select either calming or relaxing music, or music that resonates with you. You may resonate with music that has you singing along or swaying to help the baby into a good position. Or you may need music that has a calming effect on you. The choice is yours, and there is no right or wrong music. You could put together a playlist of both types of music.

The labour environment

The place you choose for your baby's birth will profoundly affect how you feel during labour and how your body reacts. You have an instinctive need for safety and privacy as you give birth, and achieving the best environment is very important for a safe, quick and relatively comfortable labour. *Preparing For Birth: Partners* includes suggestions for setting up the labour environment at the hospital or home.

The people you choose to be with you during labour and birth will also play a significant role in you staying calm and unworried. You will need to decide where to give birth and which caregiver will best meet your needs.

Extra support people

Research has shown that a known companion's continuous presence can significantly shorten labour and reduce the need for painkilling drugs. While many women feel they only want their partner with them during labour, both you and your partner may benefit from an extra pair of hands (or two!) to help provide physical assistance with massage and positional support. Being able to call on an assistant to help with these physical tasks means that the labouring woman has the comfort she needs at all times.

An extra support person can also provide the labouring woman and her partner with emotional support and physical energy. The additional person can take over some of the mundane jobs such as getting drinks and rubbing backs so that the couple can enjoy the emotional experience of giving birth together.

Choosing an extra support person

When you are considering whom to invite, choose someone whom you both know well and in whose presence you feel comfortable. You may like another woman's emotional support (especially if she has had a baby herself). Your extra support person could be a relative, friend or doula.

> **A birth doula is a person employed to provide continuous support to a woman and her partner in the labour and shortly after birth.**

Ensure that this extra person is available and their role is clearly defined before labour begins. The additional support person must be aware you may need them to leave the birth room if you find you need some privacy. Don't invite someone who just wants to observe the birth. If you feel observed, your labour may slow (see hormones of birth on pages 21-22). You want your extra support person to be actively engaged in supporting you. Your extra support person may like to attend your birth and parenting workshops or see some videos, especially if they have never seen a baby born.

Tip: Don't feel pressured by family or friends asking to attend your birth. This is your birth and you need your ideal support team.

Positions of your baby at term

During your antenatal visits, the midwife or doctor will examine your tummy to determine the baby's position. Ask your caregiver to explain the baby's position. You may be able to work this out for yourself by judging where you feel the most activity.

The way your baby is lying at the end of your pregnancy may influence the kind of labour you have and how the baby is born. A woman with a baby in the posterior position rather than in an anterior position may have a longer labour. The majority of breech babies are born by caesarean.

Anterior

The baby's back is facing towards the mother's front. The anterior position is the most favourable position for birth.

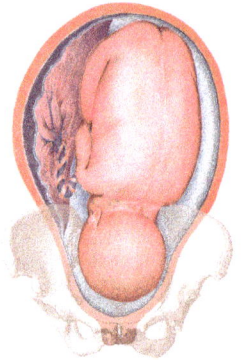

Lateral

The baby's back is facing towards the mother's side. During labour, this baby will usually turn anterior. Lateral is the most common position for a baby to be in at the start of labour.

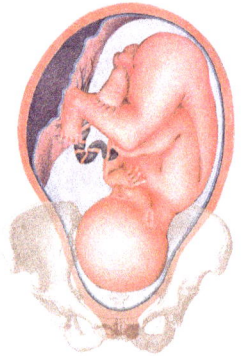

Posterior

The baby's back is facing towards the mother's spine. This position occurs in approximately 30% of all pregnancies at term. During labour, the baby usually turns to an anterior position to be born. Occasionally (about 5 to 8% of all births), the baby does not turn and is born with the face towards the mother's pubic bone.

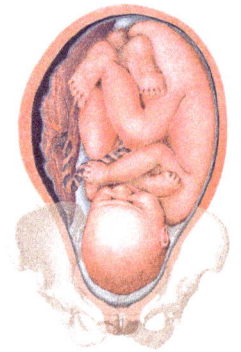

Breech

Only about 3 to 4% of babies lie in this position.

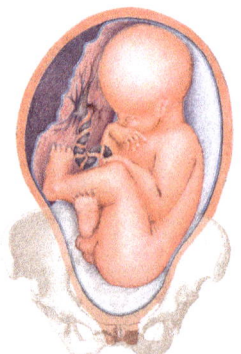

If your baby is breech

Most breech babies will turn naturally before labour. However, to increase the chance of this happening, there are several things you can try.

Positioning

If the baby settles (engages) into the pelvis, it will be difficult for the baby to turn. The following exercises, done five to seven times a day, holding for 30 to 60 seconds, may help discourage the baby from settling into the pelvis. Talk to your midwife or doctor before commencing any positioning exercise.

To do this forward-leaning inversion, use a low lounge or a piece of furniture suitable for kneeling. With the aid of your partner or support person supporting your shoulders, slowly and carefully place one hand and then the other on the ground. Walk your hands one pace forward and then go down on one forearm and then the other as in the illustration.

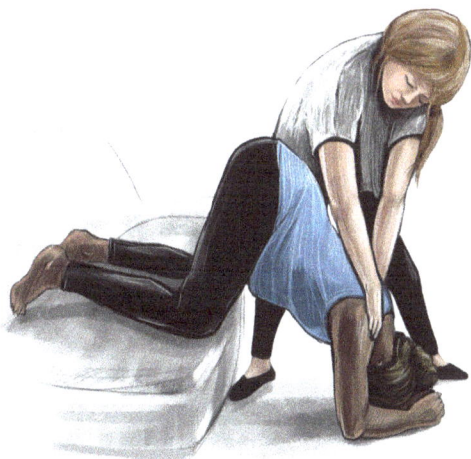

As an alternative, adopt a 'knee-chest' position, with your bottom high in the air and head and chest resting on the floor. Note the angle of the legs in the image. To help you maintain this position, have your feet resting against a piece of furniture or another person. Have your partner or a support person stand between your shoulders and head (this stops you from sliding forward).

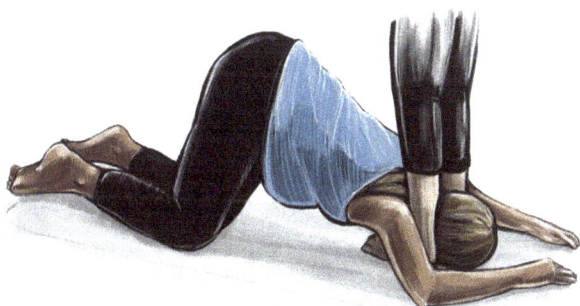

External cephalic version

Research indicates that manually massaging the baby into a better position is often successful for turning breech babies if done around 37 to 39 weeks. You will need to find a caregiver skilled in this procedure, and they may offer you a medication to stop the uterus's painless contractions while attempting to move the baby's position. There is a very slight risk that the cord will be entangled or the placenta starts to separate as the baby turns. Doing an external cephalic version in a hospital is ideal, where a caesarean is available in the unlikely event of an emergency.

Complementary therapies

Using acupuncture and acupressure may encourage babies to turn from a breech position. You will need to find a skilled practitioner to assist you.

Using the heat from burning 'moxa' sticks can also stimulate the baby and encourage it to turn. These sticks, shaped like cigars, are available from herbalists. You'll need two sticks, and they are suitable for multiple uses. Sit on a chair and place each foot on a book with your little toes hanging over the edge. Place each stick on another book with the tip in the gap. Light the sticks (they burn with no flame but intense heat and pungent smell) and position the hot end as close as possible to the outside of each little toe, with the heat directed at the point just above the toenail. Leave in place for 15 to 20 minutes.

Do moxibustion just before bed, starting at 34–36 weeks. It takes several hours for the baby to turn, which will be easier if you are lying down. Continue over several nights or until the baby has turned itself.

The research indicates that more babies will be head down at birth using moxibustion in pregnancy compared to not using moxibustion. If the baby persists in a breech position, an external cephalic version is an option before labour begins.

Giving birth to a breech baby

Often caesarean birth is recommended for a breech baby due to safety. However, research shows that a vaginal birth is a safe option if a skilled midwife or doctor is available. Many breech babies can be born safely vaginally in hospital. The risk of caesarean birth to the mother may outweigh any potential risk to the baby from vaginal birth.

Shop around for a caregiver if your baby is breech. Consider their experience in performing external cephalic version and a willingness to support vaginal birth.

If your baby is in a posterior position

During the last weeks of pregnancy, most babies will adopt a position with their back towards the side or front of their mother's tummy. However, a significant number of babies adopt a position where their back is lying near the mother's spine, in a 'posterior position'.

The assumption is that the modern lifestyle, which is often more sedentary than in the past, may be an underlying cause of the increasing number of babies lying in a posterior position at the start of labour. Your baby may be lying in this position if you notice:

- the baby's kicks being felt at the front of your tummy rather than at the side
- you have chronic backache, especially in the last weeks
- the baby does not engage (settle) into the pelvis in the last weeks of the pregnancy
- the membranes rupture at the end of pregnancy with no immediate contractions.

Encourage your baby into a good position

You can encourage your baby to align itself into the most favourable position for labour by trying the following suggestions:

- Sit upright or lean forward rather than in a reclining position when you are working and relaxing. These positions will be more comfortable as they will remove pressure from your lower spine and enable gravity to help swing your baby away from the posterior position.
- Sit back to front on a straight-backed kitchen chair or use a birth ball for easy mobilising. Avoid sitting with your feet up, reclining back into a lounge chair when relaxing and lying on your back.
- Do some moderate exercise each day, such as walking or swimming. The natural pelvic rocking that occurs when exercising will encourage your baby to move into a favourable position.
- If you have backache in later pregnancy, leaning forward and circling your hips or 'belly dancing' can help relieve the pain and encourage the baby to turn away from your spine. See page 17 for ideas.
- You can engage your partner or support person into using a rebozo. A rebozo is a traditional Mexican shawl used to sift or jiggle a baby into a better position (refer to *Preparing for Birth: Partners* for using a rebozo).

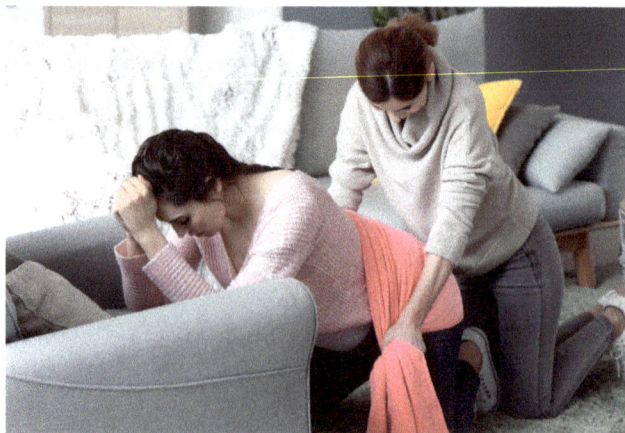

During labour

Posterior labour is often long and painful, as it takes extra time for the baby to turn before being born. Pain occurs from the pressure of the baby's head against nerves in the lower back. The pain is experienced in between the contractions, as well as during them. However, these factors will cause additional endorphins to be released, which enable you to manage this kind of labour. The support of your partner and the midwife is vital.

You can help yourself with the following suggestions:

- Choose a forward-leaning, well-supported position for labour, preferably using a mat on the floor. You need to feel safe and to have complete freedom to move around as necessary.
- Ask your partner or support person to do sacral massage.

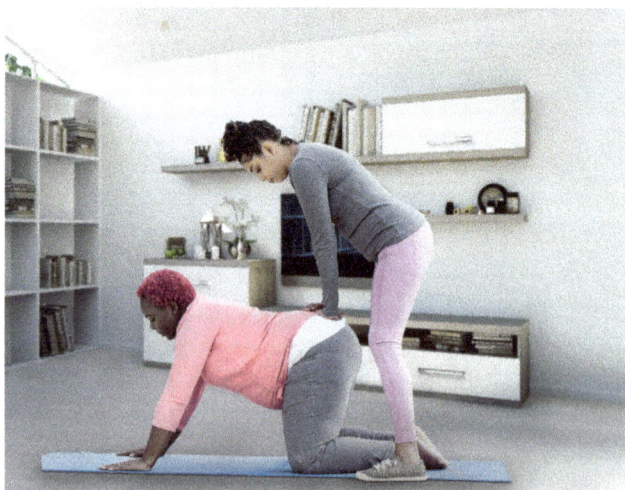

- Use water and heat (shower, bath or hot, wet towels) to ease the pain in your back.
- Stay quiet and focused. This labour is normal but will be longer than most.
- Drink fluids regularly.
- Empty your bladder every two hours to create space for the baby.

- Walk up and down some stairs to encourage the baby to move.
- Encourage your support team to take regular breaks, including naps, so they remain energised. You may need to arrange for additional supporters to take turns with your partner.

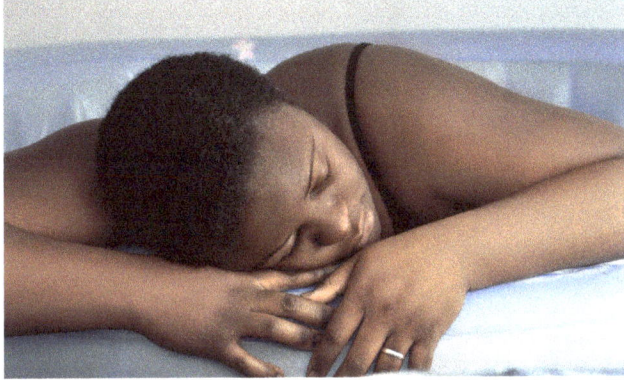

Caregivers may offer women an epidural if they make a diagnosis of posterior labour. An epidural, while it will usually ease the pain, has disadvantages. Refer to page 57 to read more about epidurals.

Giving birth without help brings particular rewards. Your baby will benefit from the additional endorphins you can produce and will usually be healthy and ready to breastfeed immediately. The sense of achievement and euphoria that you may feel will help balance the memory of the hard work you have undertaken to birth your baby.

Preparing for labour

Avoiding a perineal tear

The perineum is the area between the vagina and anus. This area stretches as the baby is born, and a tear may result. In some cases, a midwife or doctor may recommend an episiotomy where a cut is made in the vaginal opening (see page 59 for further information). A tear is common, and most heal well. However, some tears can be severe, and you can do the following steps to reduce the risk of this happening:

- talk to your midwife or doctor about tears and episiotomies, so you are informed
- start perineal massage from 34 weeks (see next section)
- pelvic floor exercises in pregnancy may reduce the chance of a severe tear (see page 59)
- a warm compress applied to your perineum as the baby is born significantly reduces the incidence of severe tearing

- research shows perineal massage with oil by your midwife or doctor as the baby is born may reduce severe tears. However, you may not like anyone touching your perineum as you are giving birth. This option is not for everyone.

Perineal massage

From 34 weeks of pregnancy, massaging the perineal area will increase the tissues's elasticity in this area and accustom you to the second stage's stretching sensations as the baby's head emerges. Research shows that perineal massage helps reduce the risk of a tear occurring or the need for an episiotomy. You only need to do perineal massage two to three times per week (doing it more often doesn't improve outcomes). Follow the steps below:

- Begin by lying back and using a mirror to locate the vagina, and the perineum, between the vaginal opening and the anus. Using a natural vegetable oil on your thumbs, insert them three to four centimetres inside the vagina and press the perineum towards the rectum and sides. If you and your partner are comfortable with this, then your partner can assist with the massage.
- Gently stretch the opening until you feel a slight burning or tingling. Maintain pressure for two minutes until the area becomes a little numb. Then slowly massage in the oil, maintaining the stretch and pressure.
- Massage for three to four minutes, concentrating on any previous episiotomy scars, which will be especially inelastic.
- According to your preference, perineal massage can also be done with a sweeping motion from side to side, with fingers moving together in one direction or opposite directions.

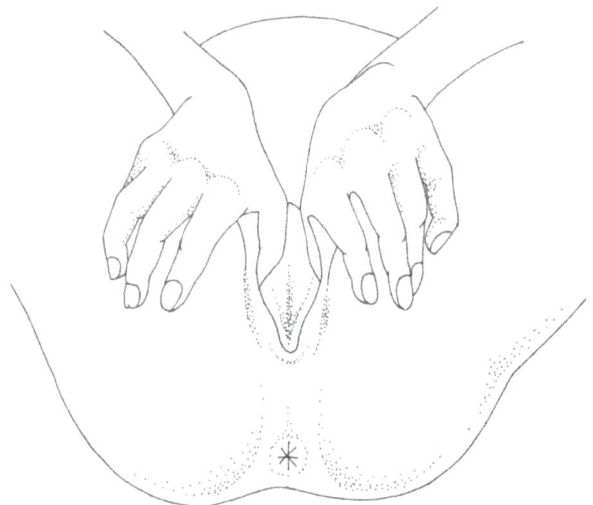

Making the most of your pelvis

Your pelvis makes a bony cradle for your baby during the pregnancy. In labour, the baby must move through this bony cradle to be born and to help make this easy, nature assists in several ways.

The pregnancy hormones help to soften ligaments around joints, making the joints in the pelvis (the pubic joint at the front and the sacroiliac joints on each side of the spine) more flexible and supple. By assuming an upright posture, leaning forward and taking weight on your open legs, you can increase your pelvis's internal size by about 28%. Upright posture is helpful in making the birth quicker, easier and less painful.

The design of the bones in a baby's head allows them to over-ride each other slightly as the head moves through the pelvis in labour. The overriding bones make the baby's head smaller in diameter and help it fit readily through the pelvis. The skin on the baby's head will become loose if the head moulds in this way, and as it is being born, the scalp may look like a wrinkled walnut! The bones will resume their normal position within a day or two, and your baby's head will have a rounded shape once more.

Gravity will assist these two processes of moulding and opening of the pelvis. To take full advantage of gravity, you need to be in an upright position to ensure the acting forces are in the right direction. See the labour section for some advantageous positions.

You can help avoid forceps to lift the baby out by using gravity. Even if you are tired and find pushing hard, gravity, together with your uterine contractions, is often enough to help birth your baby. You'll need to be well supported and in a favourable, upright position.

Deciding on your birth preferences

There are many options and possibilities for labour and birth. You may have attended the birth and parenting classes, read some books, seen some videos, and talked to your friends. Therefore you'll have some ideas of what you might like during labour and birth. You'll also know those things you would like to avoid.

To help you clarify your ideas, the list below offers many possible options. Hospitals vary enormously in the services they provide and the routines they use to manage labour.

In many places, you will be encouraged to labour as you wish, and the issues listed below won't arise. However, don't rely on this – it is better to have discussed your ideas in advance than to be disappointed later when your preferences run counter to prevailing hospital routines and protocols.

Assume the pregnancy, labour and birth will be normal unless there are clear medical indications that a problem has occurred. Go through the list, tick the options you would like and put a cross against those you don't want or are unsure about.

During the pregnancy

Choice of caregiver

- ○ Private midwife
- ○ Hospital-based midwife
- ○ General practitioner
- ○ Obstetrician
- ○ Shared care by midwife or doctor

Place of birth

- ○ Birth centre
- ○ Home
- ○ Hospital maternity unit

Labour

- ○ Wearing own clothes
- ○ Electronic fetal monitoring test trace on admission
- ○ Consent to be a teaching patient (students and staff present at any time)
- ○ Returning home if not in established labour
- ○ Food/fluids on request throughout labour
- ○ Intravenous drip in labour
- ○ External fetal monitoring throughout labour
- ○ Internal fetal monitoring
- ○ Monitoring fetal heart rate by hand (fetal doppler)
- ○ Freedom to choose positions and activity in labour (walking, sitting, squatting, kneeling, etc.)
- ○ Vaginal exam for specific medical indication only
- ○ Complete information on the risks and benefits of each suggested medical procedure
- ○ Artificial rupture of the membranes
- ○ Artificial hormone (oxytocin) to boost contractions or induce labour
- ○ Access to the water pool, shower or bath for pain relief
- ○ Analgesia or anaesthesia for pain in labour: Kind preferred ....
- ○ Partner/chosen person(s) present at all times
- ○ Siblings present for labour
- ○ Presence of interpreter

Birth

- O Presence of partner/chosen person(s) during the actual birth
- O Your child/ren present for the birth
- O Partner/chosen person(s) present for caesarean birth
- O Position for the second stage selected by mother
- O Pushing begun on mother's urge only
- O Anaesthesia for delivery:
  Kind preferred ....
- O So long as making progress, no specific time limit on the second stage of labour
- O Episiotomy
- O Freedom to touch baby during birth
- O Partner/mother assisting with actual birth by hand
- O Midwife to assist baby's birth
- O Female rather than a male doctor
- O Baby allowed to take first breaths unassisted (no immediate suctioning, etc.)
- O Late cord clamping (after pulsating stops)
- O Skin-to-skin contact for mother and partner with the baby immediately after birth
- O Artificial hormone injection (oxytocin) after the birth to expel the placenta
- O Baby on the breast to stimulate expulsion of placenta
- O Vernix left on
- O The baby weighed, measured in parents' presence after the initial bonding period

Postnatal

- O Baby remains with mother at all times (nights included)
- O Person of choice in mother's room at any time of day
- O Breastfeeding on demand from birth
- O Help with breastfeeding on request
- O Formula feeding
- O Vitamin K for baby: oral/injection/withheld unless requested by parents
- O Hepatitis B vaccination for the baby
- O Circumcision
- O Early discharge from hospital as soon as mother wishes

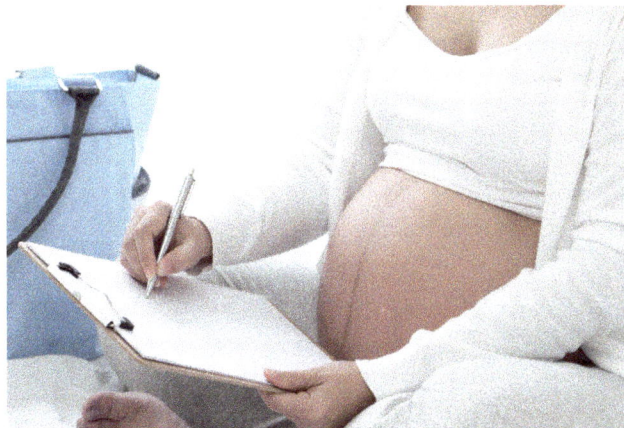

Implementing your birth preferences

It may not be easy to have the birth experience you have planned. Caregivers and hospitals vary in their views and practices, and it is wise to work out your particular requirements early in the pregnancy so you can take steps to find the services you will need in plenty of time for the birth. Options for caregivers and birthplaces have been explained in *Preparing For Birth: Partners*. You will want to discuss these ideas in detail with your partner or support person and enlist their help in negotiating with hospital staff and caregivers. Remember that this is your birth, so you have the right to accept or decline interventions or recommendations after gathering information to inform yourself.

Here are some ideas on how you can achieve your goals:

- Find out as much as you can about birth: the process, current practices in hospitals, professional views, etc. Don't just rely on what your friends experienced; ask around widely. Your educator will have plenty of information too.
- When you feel ready to make decisions, use the birth preference list above to help work out what is important to you. Some aspects you may or may not want. In some areas, you may not have strong feelings.
- Discuss your needs with the midwife or doctor as soon as possible. Determine which areas may need further discussion or compromise and those areas in which you agree.
- Visit the hospital and find out their procedures and how they can meet your needs. Decide if there are areas where compromise will be needed.
- Think about these areas needing compromise. How important are these issues to you? Can you think of any solutions that may be acceptable to all parties?
- Discuss your ideas further with the midwife or doctor and hospital staff. Try to work out mutually acceptable compromises in the areas in which you feel this is needed.
- Look again at your chosen caregiver and birthplace: are there any others who might be willing to accommodate your needs where compromise won't be needed?
- If you feel you can achieve a happier result with another caregiver or hospital, then consider changing. You can do this even late in pregnancy if you want, and your new caregiver will request your medical notes from your previous one (you could also request these notes yourself).

- If you don't want to change caregivers, you have two choices: you can stand your ground on your preferences or accommodate their wishes in certain areas. By deciding early in pregnancy, there will be more time to negotiate your care.
- Ensure that both the midwife or doctor and the hospital staff know, well in advance of your labour, what you would like. Revisit the hospital if necessary to finalise arrangements with the birth unit staff and the postnatal staff. You could also ask your caregiver for a letter outlining the care you want to take with you to the hospital. This way, even if they don't make it or arrive late in labour, you have a chance of getting the experience you have planned. Make sure that this letter is attached to your medical notes.

It is important to remember the following information when going through these steps:

- Your caregiver might not be willing to change their method of managing births to accommodate your wishes. You might be better off seeking a more sympathetic person who practises more in line with your wishes.
- If you have a request that is not usual practice at the hospital, contact them to negotiate a care plan. They may be unable to provide your ideal care if not prewarned that you will want it.
- The most crucial point of all: caregivers cannot read your mind. Talk to the midwife or doctor about anything that is bothering you. Don't assume that all will be well. Make sure you ask and check with them. Then everyone knows where they stand.

BRAIN decision-making tool

Using the BRAIN decision-making tool can help you navigate pregnancy and birth decisions. Which tests and procedures do you want? How should your birth preferences look? These are opportunities to make proactive choices for yourself and your baby.

The BRAIN acronym helps you remember what questions to ask at antenatal appointments, write your birth plan, and make decisions on recommendations while in labour. Here is an outline of the BRAIN decision-making tool.

Benefits

What are the benefits of the suggested course of action? Consider benefits to both you and your baby.

Risks

Consider the risks associated with this decision. Any side effects? Remember that different people will weigh the advantages and disadvantages differently. Remember that what's important to you might not be to someone else.

Alternatives

Are there other options available?

Intuition

How do I feel about the suggested course of action? Our subconscious quietly analyses the information in a way that our conscious brain can't. If nothing else, acknowledging your feelings makes them easier to process.

Nothing

Consider the implications if I do nothing? What if we wait for an hour, a day or a week?

You might need to ask your midwife or doctor for time to decide, even just 10 minutes alone may help.

Following the birth

After the birth, you may like to implement the following suggestions:

- Write to the hospital and midwife or doctor and thank them for their care, particularly any 'extras' provided. This feedback will let them know that you were happy with their efforts, but it helps encourage them to be open to others who will follow you.
- If you are unhappy about some aspect of your care, tell the appropriate people that too. They need to know how you felt about their assistance.
- Attend your birth and parenting course reunion, if there is one, and let your classmates know how you went and give your educator some feedback.

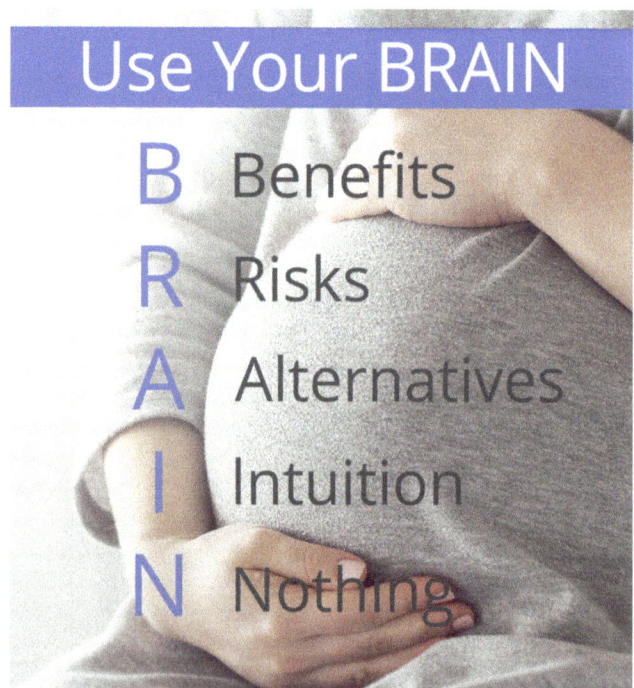

Use Your BRAIN

B Benefits
R Risks
A Alternatives
I Intuition
N Nothing

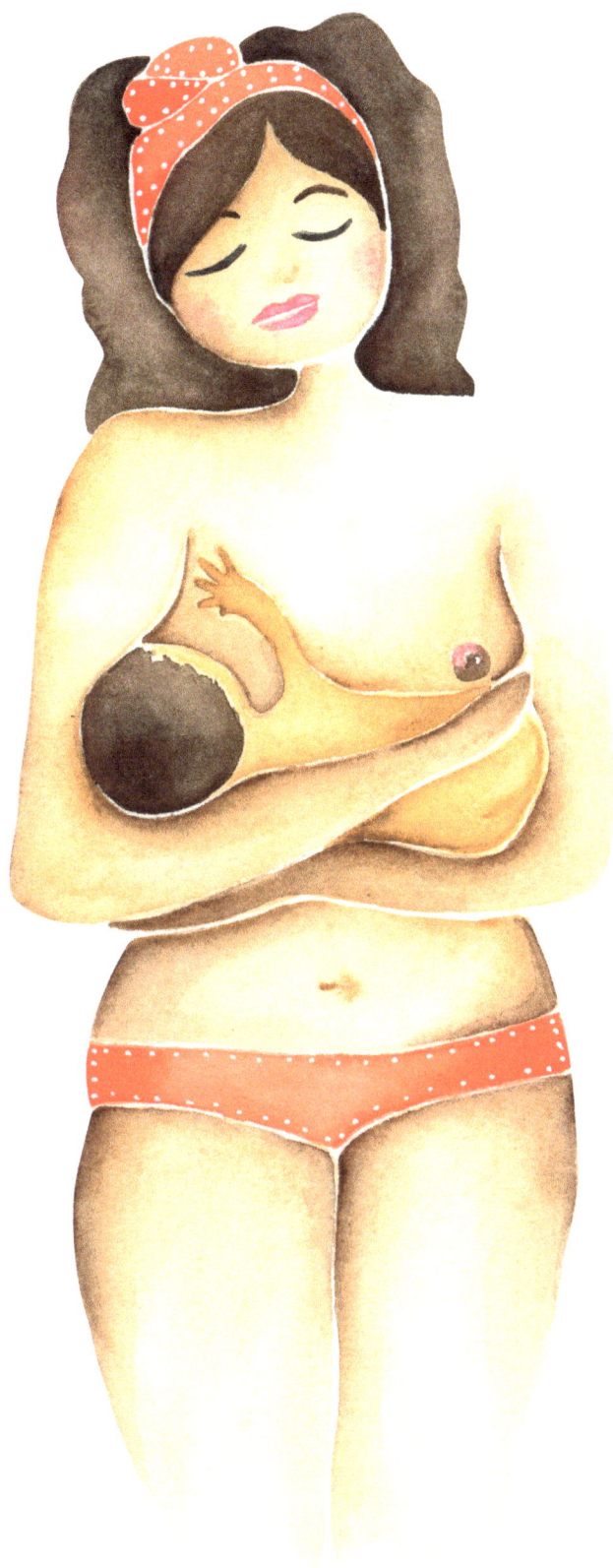

The birth of your baby

Labour begins

Signs of impending labour

In the last weeks of pregnancy, you may notice some of the following signs that your body and the baby are getting ready for labour:

- the baby's head engages in the pelvis. Engagement happens two to six weeks before labour begins but may not occur until labour starts (especially if this is not your first baby)
- Braxton-Hicks contractions: usually painless tightenings of the uterus, but occurring more often than in the earlier months of pregnancy, perhaps as 'sets' of contractions
- increased mucous discharge from the vagina
- you experience a spurt of energy, known as nesting behaviour
- slight diarrhoea
- pelvic pressure as the baby's position is low in the pelvis
- a 'show' of pink mucous discharge from the vagina, perhaps streaked with blood
- waters breaking with no subsequent labour contractions.

How will you know you are in labour?

Following some of the signs listed above, contractions will develop. These feel different from the Braxton-Hicks contractions of pregnancy. Labour contractions:

- have a rhythmic quality, with each one gradually building to a peak and then fading
- develop into a pattern of increasing intensity over time. The length of time between each one is less significant than the contraction's length and strength
- require concentration. You won't want to talk or continue with daily activities
- encourage you to find a comfortable position to ease the pain
- are strong enough that you will want to rest in between them
- are sometimes felt like a constant minor backache, with regular bouts of more substantial back pain.

Until the contractions are feeling like this, you are probably not in labour.

Occasionally, the membranes leak or break before labour (in about 6–19% of cases). If your waters break, put on a pad, check the colour of the water and note the time. Then call your midwife, doctor or hospital. Contractions may start immediately, but often they take hours or even days to become established.

When to go to hospital

During the first part of labour, you will be most comfortable at home, in a familiar environment where you can make yourself comfortable. As the contractions become more productive, they will begin to settle into a pattern. The best guide to the intensity and strength of contractions is their length, and once they last 60 seconds or more consistently, dilatation will occur.

You will know when you feel you need to go to the hospital, and as soon as you no longer feel comfortable in your home, you should ask your partner to take you. It is wise to stay at home as long as possible to avoid unnecessary hours in the hospital, especially for your first baby. Make sure you ring the hospital first before heading in.

When you get to the hospital, go to the admission desk and complete the formalities. You will be shown to the birth unit by a staff member.

If you have a homebirth, you will naturally stay at home and call the midwife when you want them to be with you. In the unlikely event of a complication, your midwife will indicate when it's appropriate to go to the hospital.

> **If labour begins before 37 weeks, contact your midwife, doctor or hospital right away as your baby may be born prematurely.**

Admission into hospital

When you arrive in the birth unit, the midwife will take basic observations such as blood pressure, urine check, temperature, obstetric history, pregnancy history. The midwife will then listen to the baby's heartbeat and feel its position in the abdomen. The midwife may offer an internal examination to assess progress, although this is not compulsory. You can sit on a chair or stand supported by your partner for these examinations.

Some hospitals have a policy of recording a 20–30 minute trace on the electronic fetal monitor as part of their admission procedure. Evidence shows no benefit or need for routine electronic fetal monitoring if you and the baby are well. If you require monitoring, you don't need to lie down as you can sit or stand. After completion of admission procedures, the midwife will show you to your room in the birth unit.

Sometimes, labour can slow down when you get to the hospital and can even stop altogether. If this happens, it is your body's natural reaction to the change of environment. Read about the effect of adrenaline on page 22. Give yourself time to adjust to the surroundings and the staff. Labour will re-establish when you are feeling comfortable. Alternatively, you might want to go home again, especially if you are in early labour.

How long is labour?

Every mother would like to know how long her labour will be before she begins. Unfortunately, it is impossible to anticipate how long labour will take because every woman is different. In general, giving birth to your first baby takes longer than giving birth to subsequent children, but each labour will still vary. Keep an open mind, as this will help you prepare for all eventualities.

The early part of labour varies widely from woman to woman. Early labour is the time before dilation reaches four to six centimetres. It can be hours or even many days. The beginning of actual labour, known as the active first stage of labour, starts from five to six cm (definitions vary). The active first stage ends when the cervix is fully open, 10 centimetres dilation, and generally doesn't last more than 12 hours for first babies or more than 10 hours for subsequent babies.

The second stage of labour, from when the cervix reaches 10 centimetres dilation and ends with the baby's birth, takes up to three hours for first babies and up to two hours for subsequent babies.

Remember, your body knows how to give birth, just as your body knows how to grow the baby in the first place. Trust in your instincts and allow yourself time to explore the sensations you will feel. How long it will take depends on many factors, such as your comfort, emotional support, the position of the baby, the position you assume and how you feel about becoming a mother. Having a baby is an adventure into the unknown but an enormously rewarding one.

The Journey of Labour

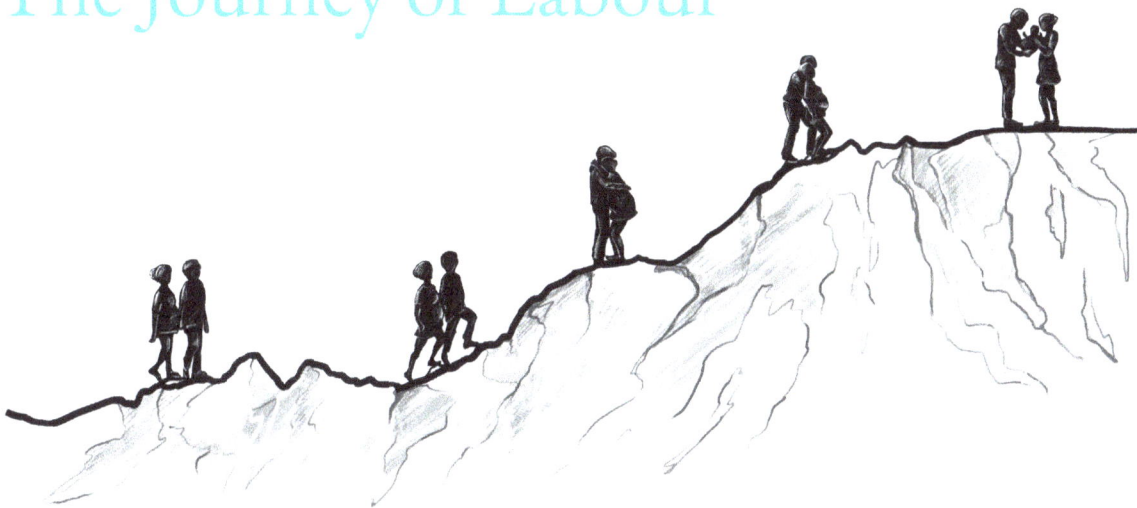

~ Everyone's journey is different ~

Early Labour	Active Labour	Transition	Birth	Placenta's Arrival
Beginning the journey	Starts around the time the cervix opening is 5 to 6cm	Occurs before the second phase of labour	Cervix is fully open	Forgotten phase
Excitement	Strong	Transitioning from one phase to the next	Home stretch	Baby is born
Unpredictable	Intense	Tumultuous	Baby is almost here	Skin to skin
May stop and start	Hard work	Overwhelming	Joy	Cramping
May be short or long	Space between contractions decreases	May need extra support	Relief	Backache
Pain mild to strong	Length of most contractions increases to 60 seconds or more	Contractions back to back with often little break between	Pushing	Pressure
Spacing between contractions varies		Generally lasts a few contractions to 1.5 hours	Contractions more spaced apart	Important part of birth
May be more challenging than anticipated			Burning sensation as the baby emerges	

It is often difficult to pinpoint when labour has begun as there can be quite a long period in which some early labour signs are present, but little other action (see the journey of labour image on the previous page). There are many variations on this theme, and you will have to wait until the contractions start to discover how your body will undertake the task of giving birth. You may need the close support of your partner or support person or you may want to journey alone. Be prepared to accept whatever your particular labour brings and allow yourself time to adjust and to appreciate the powerful energy that is yours as you give birth.

Making labour easier with active birth

Active birth is where you work with your body's ability to give birth using the right environment, support, upright positions and relaxation strategies. In general, your body will work best if you feel safe and secure as you labour and actively make choices about your care. You can make labour easier with the following suggestions:

- Organise close, continuous support from your partner, close friends or relatives during labour. Suitable support has been shown to shorten labours and reduce the need for pain medication.
- Find a place to labour in that is dark, quiet and cosy. Alter your room in the birth unit by dimming the lights and keeping the door closed. You can also move the bed to give yourself more floor space for mats, bean bags, chairs etc.
- Stay as vertical as you can to stimulate the labour and make the contractions more comfortable. The following pages show how you can assume upright positions.
- Consume regular drinks during labour and eat light snacks in the early stages.
- Stay focused on what you are doing and respond to your instinctive urges as necessary. For once in your life, you can be the complete centre of attention and have your support team fulfil your every wish.

> **Active birth is where you work with your body's ability to give birth using the right environment, support, upright positions and relaxation strategies.**

Your labour and birth

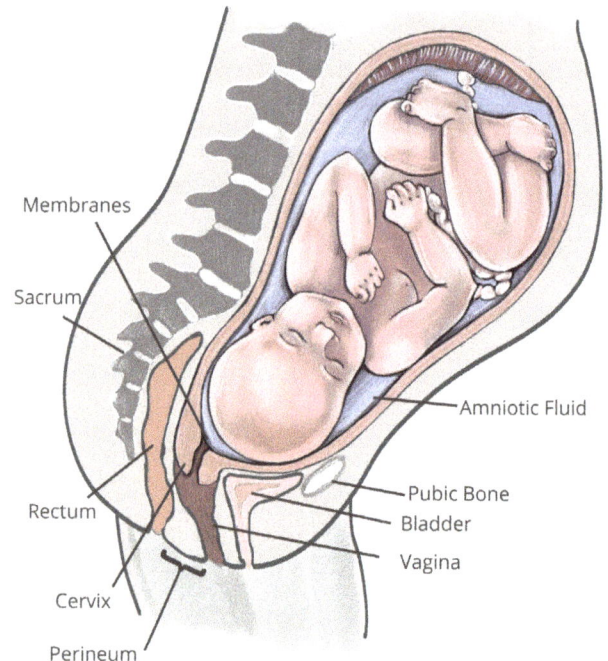

Membranes
Sacrum
Amniotic Fluid
Pubic Bone
Rectum
Bladder
Vagina
Cervix
Perineum

First stage

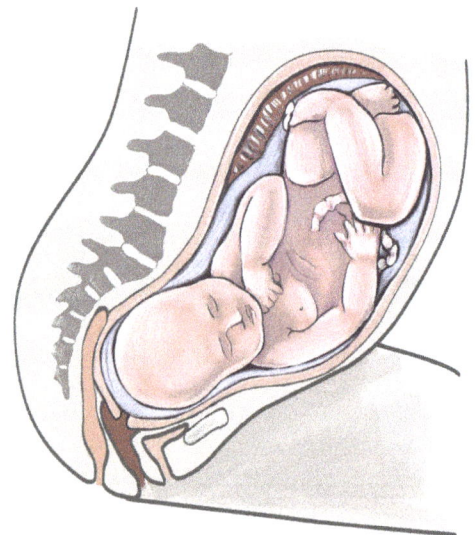

During this stage, the cervix dilates from closed to open (0–10 centimetres). The baby moves down deeper into the pelvis, and the face gradually turns towards the mother's back.

Helping yourself
If you think that labour might be about to start:

- Conserve your energy, but keep on with your usual activities if it is daytime. If labour begins at night, try to rest or sleep.

- Take a shower, go for a walk, but don't tire yourself.
- Don't skip any meals, particularly if labour starts during the night or early in the morning. Have something light, nourishing and easily digested, such as scrambled eggs, soup, tea and toast.
- Pack the car with the things you wish to take to the hospital and your labour 'goody bag'.
- Carry on with your usual daily routine until contractions become well established, and you can be sure that labour has begun.
- Contact your support people to alert them that your labour may be starting soon.

If the waters break, note the colour of the fluid. It should be clear or slightly pink. If it is yellow/brown/green, you should contact your midwife, doctor or hospital right away. If a baby does a poo inside your tummy, it causes your waters to be this colour. Sometimes this is a sign of a baby in distress.

If you begin labour before 37 weeks, you should contact your midwife, doctor or hospital right away as the baby may be born prematurely.

Early labour

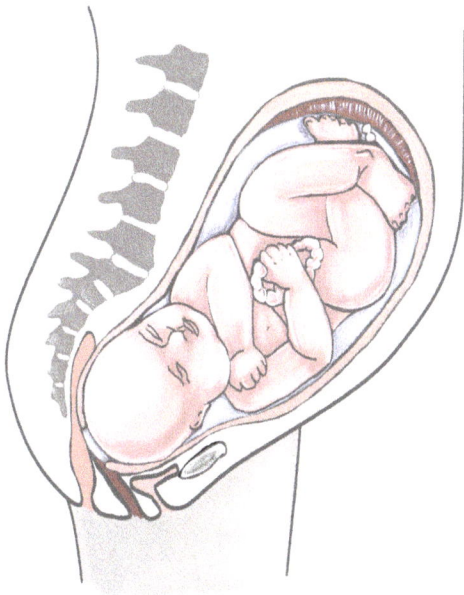

During this part of labour, the cervix softens, shortens (effaces) and begins to dilate (open up). Early labour can stop and start and can last many days.

Helping yourself
Follow the suggestions below in this stage of labour:

- The most important tip is to rest as much as possible. This part of labour can be very gradual, and you want to conserve energy for the active part of labour.

- Continue eating as long as you feel like it.
- Have regular drinks such as water or sports drinks, about one cupful every hour.
- Move around until you find a comfortable position.
- Continue light activities as long as you feel able (but don't overdo it).
- Take each contraction as it comes, deal with it, then rest up for the next one. Listen to your body and find ways of making its work easier and more comfortable.

Active labour

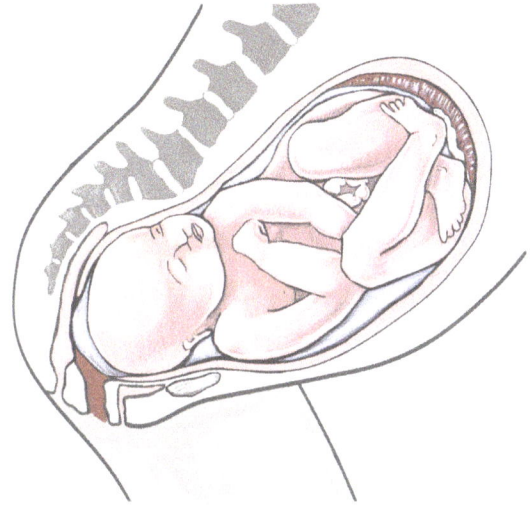

As dilatation reaches around five to six centimetres, labour enters the active phase of labour. In the active phase, your contractions will be stronger, closer together and will require concentration. Rest up between contractions. You'll start to feel more introverted and focused on what's going on within your body.

Helping yourself
Follow the suggestions below in this stage of labour:

- Conserve energy by finding positions where you can relax, fully supported, both during and between contractions.
- Keep drinking fluids or, if feeling nauseous, have sips of water or suck on ice chips.
- Ask your support people to provide massage or back rubs whenever you need them.
- In between contractions, ask support people for general massage, hot or cold packs or anything else you need to stay comfortable and relaxed. If your feet are cold, put on your woolly socks.
- If the doctor or midwife suggests trying medication, request an internal examination to determine progress before making a decision.

- A shower or bath at this time will help you to stay relaxed. Keep changing positions until you are comfortable.

Transition

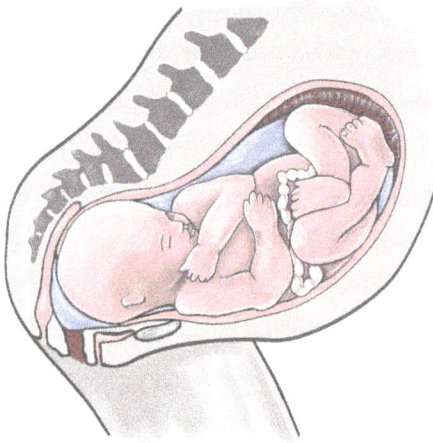

Transition is usually the most challenging part of labour. Your body is changing over from the opening up phase to the bearing down phase, and contractions are often very long (sometimes with double peaks) and close together.

It is a time of turbulent emotional feelings and announced by sudden change and feelings of being 'out of control'. If the membranes haven't ruptured earlier, this might happen during the transition, and the release of pressure may ease some of the discomforts.

Before the cervix fully dilates, there may be an urge to push. If pushing hurts at this time, then try the knee-chest position until the cervix fully dilates.

Other symptoms of transition are shivering, cramps, nausea, vomiting, hiccups. You may feel pressure on your bowel as the baby's head moves deeper into the birth canal. Transition usually lasts from a few contractions to around one and a half hours.

Helping yourself

Transition is a very turbulent time for most women. Feelings of panic, loss of control and annoying physical side-effects are all common. Your partner's support will be vital at this time, and see *Preparing For Birth: Partners* for suggestions on what they can do.

Follow the suggestions below in this stage of labour:

- You will have difficulty getting comfortable but keep changing positions. It will be hard to stay relaxed but concentrate on breathing as deeply as possible,

making some noise with each out-breath to release the tension.
- A shower or bath at this time will give excellent pain relief, but if this is not available, use your hot, wet towels to provide local relief.
- Support people need to hold, cuddle and reassure you at this time. They need to keep distractions to a minimum and concentrate on helping you through each contraction as it comes.
- Ice chips or sips of water will help dry lips and nausea.
- Cool sponges on the face and neck feel good.
- Avoid eye contact and keep your eyes closed to avoid distractions.
- If you feel the urge to push before dilatation is complete, move into the knee-chest position. Have pillows ready to lift your shoulders in between contractions.
- Reassurance and love are what you need most at this time.

Second stage

The second stage begins when your cervix is fully open. Sometimes there may be a lull between the end of the first stage and the feelings of needing to push. If this lull occurs, take the opportunity for a rest until contractions re-establish strongly. This break from contractions may last up to 30 minutes or more.

Contractions in the second stage are usually shorter than in transition and more spaced apart. Take the opportunity to rest between contractions.

Once you have the urge to push in the second stage, most babies are born within three hours with a first birth. Subsequent births are shorter, with most babies arriving within two hours of pushing in the second stage.

The urge to bear down is usually irresistible. With each pushing action, the baby moves down the birth canal. You feel pressure on the bowel as the head presses on the rectum.

As the head presses on the perineum and the vaginal tissues open out, a burning sensation will develop as the skin stretches to its maximum. This burning is a signal to push gently as the baby's head crowns, to allow a gradual stretching and easing of the skin over the baby's face.

Once the head is born, it turns to one side to line up with the shoulders. The shoulders are born one at a time, and the baby's body slips out.

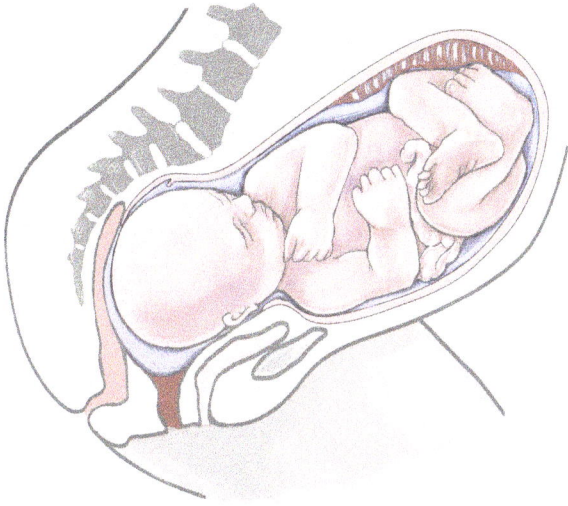
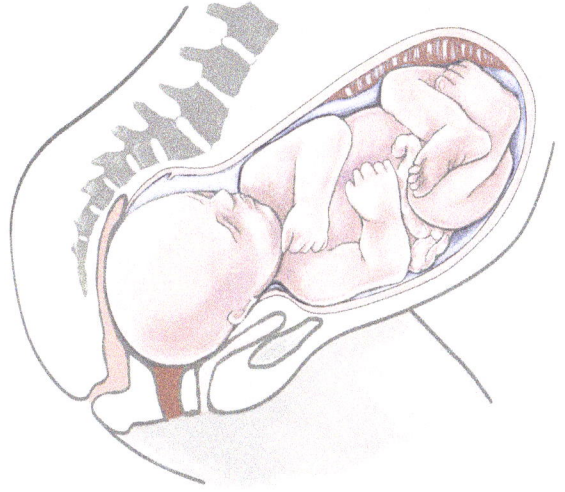
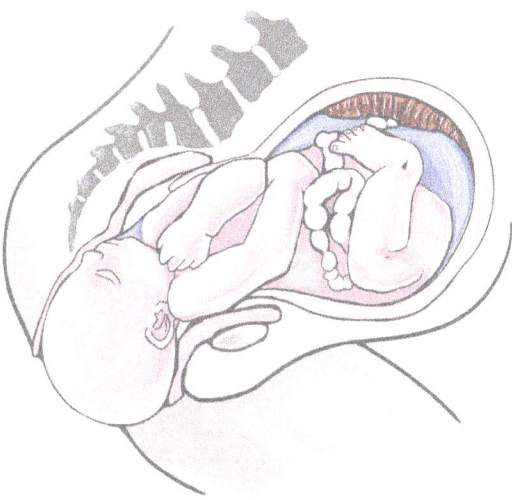
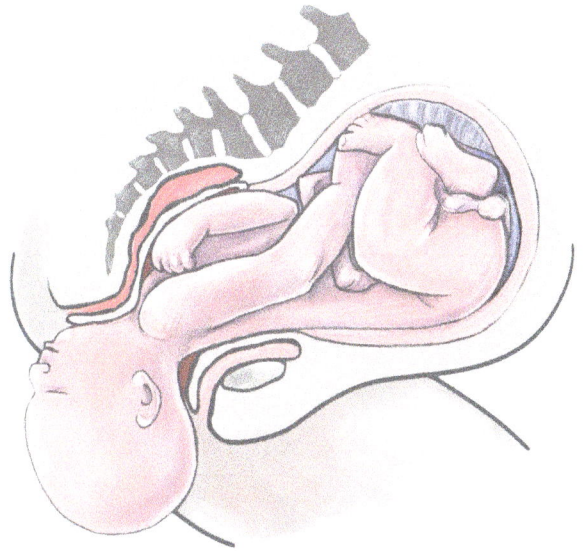
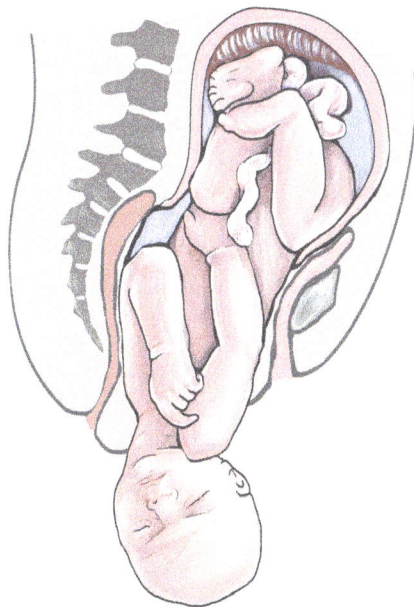

Helping yourself

Once the second stage begins, the turbulent feelings of transition will pass, and you will notice renewed energy: your second wind. Most women find pushing quite satisfying as they work with their body, and excitement is high as the moment of birth approaches.

Follow the suggestions below in this stage of labour:

- Your body dictates when and how much to push. Listen to these messages from within and concentrate on letting your body open up. Find a comfortable position for pushing with your body upright and the sacrum free to move. In between contractions, you can stand, kneel or flop forwards on to hands and knees.
- As you feel the burning sensation developing (crowning), concentrate on easing the baby out slowly. The burning sensation lasts less than a minute and will soon pass.
- Put your hand down to feel the top of the baby's head emerging from your vagina. In between contractions, rest completely and keep sipping water.

Third stage of labour

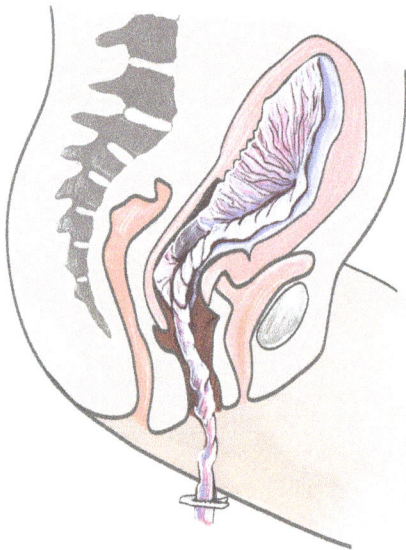

After birth, the amount of time the cord pulsates varies from three minutes up to 15 minutes or more. Once the cord stops pulsing, it can be clamped and cut either then or after the placenta has been born.

Meanwhile, the uterus shrinks in size and continues to contract, a process helped by skin to skin contact with the baby and nuzzling or sucking at the breast. The placenta begins to peel off the uterine wall and, when free, slides into the vagina. You may feel pressure in your rectum, and with pushes or just the aid of gravity, the placenta is born. The birth of the placenta, on average, takes five minutes to an hour or more. The midwife or doctor examines the placenta and membranes to ensure they are complete and that no pieces are in the uterus.

An injection of synthetic oxytocin for the third stage of labour is the policy in hospitals. Read about the use of artificial oxytocins In labour on page 51.

After the placenta's arrival, the midwife or doctor inspects your perineum for any abrasions or tears that may need some stitches. If they perform an episiotomy, the midwife or doctor will repair it.

With the baby skin-to-skin with you, everyone is left together to get to know your new baby.

Helping yourself

Follow the suggestions below in this stage of labour:

- Sit up while you are waiting for the placenta to come. Gravity helps the third stage of labour.
- Keep the room dark and warm, and keep talk to a minimum. The right flow of hormones will help you to birth the placenta.
- Skin-to-skin contact between you and the baby will help keep the baby warm, provide nipple stimulation, enhance the closeness and prevent excessive bleeding.

Using water for labour and birth

Labouring and perhaps giving birth in water offers a practical alternative for women who want to increase their comfort during labour and reduce the risks of interventions. The evidence shows that labouring in water reduces the need for pain medication, increases maternal satisfaction with the birth experience and is safe for the baby. A baby born underwater won't breathe until its face is in the air, and the change of temperature stimulates the first breath.

The options available will depend on the facilities at the chosen birthplace. It is essential to check these out well before labour. Hospitals will have policies regarding the use of the bath or pool, and many require that staff who are suitably experienced be available to assist. Having alternatives means you can decide during labour whether you want to use warm water for labour and the birth when the time comes.

If there is no bathroom in the birth room, hot, wet towels are a good substitute, and these are also very effective for easing localised pain during labour. Consider bringing an inflatable birth pool with you. Many hospitals encourage this.

If you choose to use a pool in a home setting, you'll need easy access to taps for filling, an air pump to inflate the pool, and a space to set up your birth pool. You can hire or purchase a pool for use at home. Some midwives supply an inflatable birth pool for you to use as part of their service.

Baths

Deep baths or pools take time to fill. The temperature should not be hotter than 37 degrees Celsius. A bath provides freedom of movement if large enough and enables a deep sense of calm which can lower anxiety, blood pressure and pain. They are safe to use after the membranes have broken.

Inflatable birth pool

Inflatable birth pools are designed for birth with the correct height and come with a liner for easy cleanup. Most have handles ideal for holding on to in labour. The best feature is an inflatable bottom that is very comfortable to lean on.

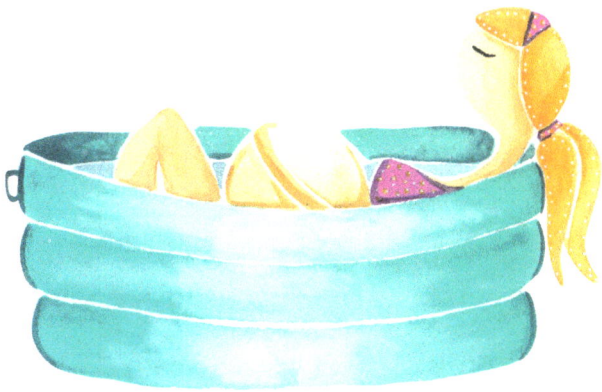

Lying or kneeling in a bath or pool encourages faster dilation.

Showers

Showers offer the advantage of immediate availability and space for your partner to support you through contractions. The temperature is not critical. Direct the water to specific areas of pain. Using the shower during transition is especially helpful when a quick change of scene and non-drug help for acute pain is helpful. Use a birth stool, a birth ball (on a folded towel) or a plastic chair for additional support. Hand-held showers work best.

Standing or sitting in the shower will help ease much of the pain, especially towards the end of the first stage.

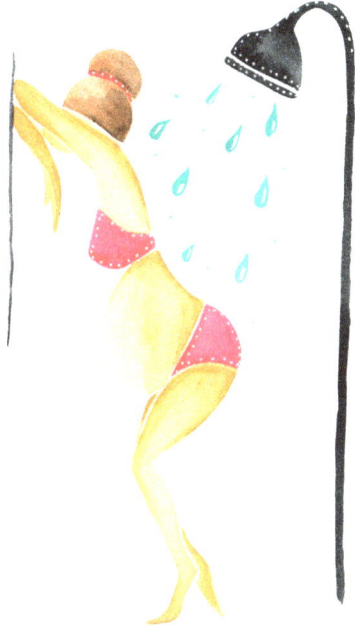

Hot wet towels

If a bath or shower is not available, using hot, wet towels can provide a helpful alternative. See *Preparing for Birth: Partners* for instructions on how to do hot, wet towels. Using hand towels wrung out in hot water and applied to local sore areas effectively relieves pain and provides a good alternative if a shower or bath is not available. Apply a fresh towel for every contraction. Use piping hot water in a bucket to heat the towels, and use rubber gloves when wringing them out.

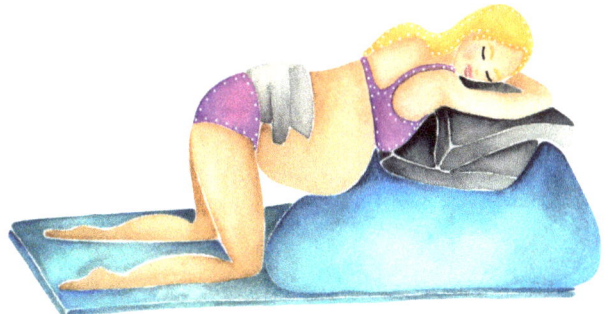

Use well wrung-out hot, wet towels draped over the buttocks for lower back pain.

Packing for birth

There are many ways of increasing your comfort during labour. Making preparations in advance will increase your confidence in helping yourself and enable you to take care of your own needs without relying on the hospital staff. Being well-equipped and knowledgeable about self-help strategies will also reduce your need for painkilling drugs.

Your 'goody bag'

Here are some suggestions for items to include in your 'goody bag'. All have proven helpful for women in labour. Consider each one, and make your list. Add any extras of your own after considering the following suggestions:

- an old t-shirt or loose button-up top to wear
- several pairs of panties and some sanitary pads – to catch leaking fluid
- thongs (flip flops) or slip-on shoes for walking around the birth unit
- your pillow(s)
- the duvet from your bed
- water bottle – to drink every hour during labour
- sports drinks or lollies for energy
- unscented massage oil
- essential oils and a diffuser
- battery-operated candles
- spray bottle to cool you down
- handheld fan
- face cloth – for wiping sweaty foreheads
- warm socks – feet get very cold in labour!
- lip balm – for dry lips
- four hand towels, rubber gloves and bucket – to make hot towels for relief of pain anywhere. The gloves should be large enough for the support person to wear. Use the bucket to carry some items from your 'goody bag' list
- tennis balls – provide firm local pressure
- food and drinks – for your support people to keep their energy up
- swimsuit or change of clothes for your support person – for use in the shower
- phone with music and earphones for music or Bluetooth speaker – to block out the world and focus on labour
- phone or camera – to record the event
- this book – to remind you of positions for labour and helpful ideas for any problems
- TENS machine
- rebozo

- positive affirmations and Blu Tack
- heat pack – either a rice bag or microwavable gel pack (check hospital policy)
- charge cords and headphones
- hair clips and ties
- snacks.

My 'goody bag' list:

....

....

....

....

....

....

....

....

....

....

Positions for labour – first stage

On the following pages are some suggestions for positions you may find helpful during labour. Experiment with these in pregnancy to find those that seem most comfortable, but be prepared to try them all again when labour is underway. In choosing the most comfortable position, remember:

- You should be as fully supported as possible, using people, pillows, bean bags or furniture to relax fully.
- Knees should be bent to avoid tiredness in the legs and to make pelvic rocking easier.
- Your feet should be apart to give a broad base for support and encourage 'open' positions.
- Be creative in your adaptation of available furniture in the hospital. If you need extra pillows or a stool or chair, request these.
- Once you find a comfortable position, use it until it is no longer helping you relax. Change positions only as you need, unless you are positioning for a specific purpose, such as assisting the baby in turning from the posterior position or encouraging the baby to move down further into the pelvis.

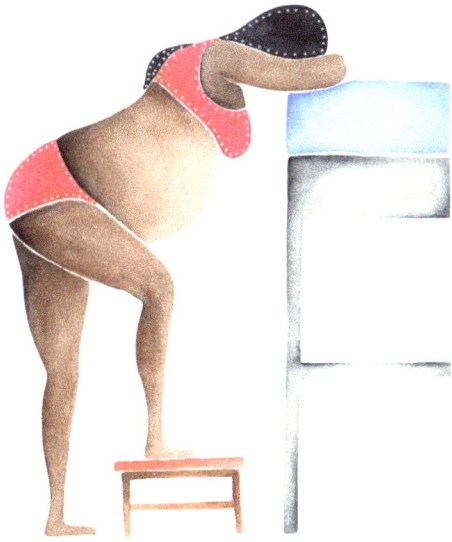

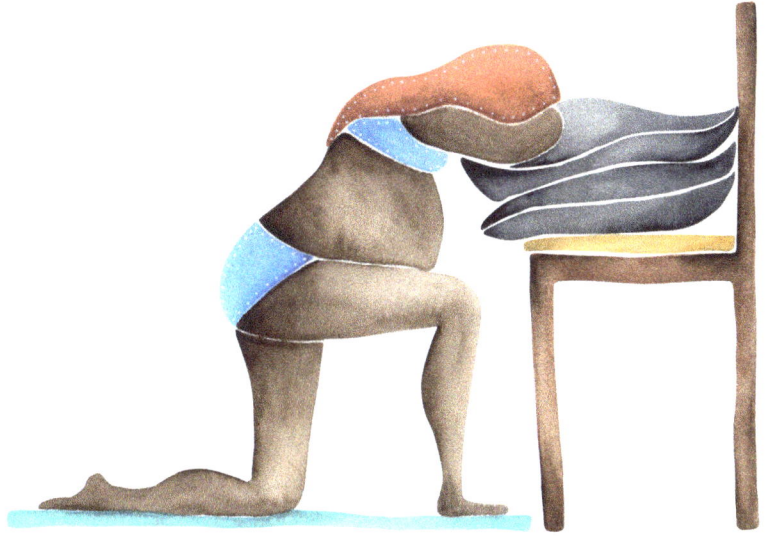

You may find asymmetrical positions help ease pressure points.

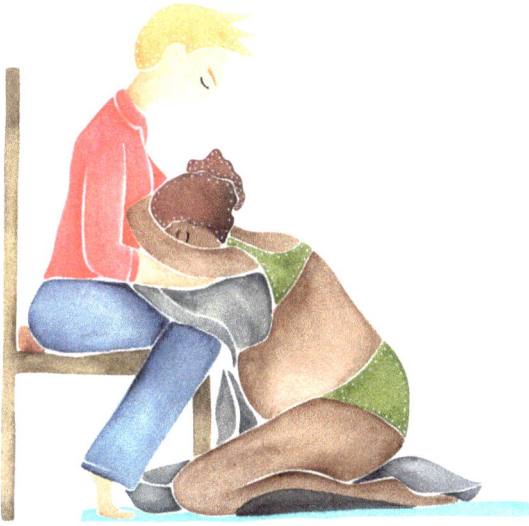

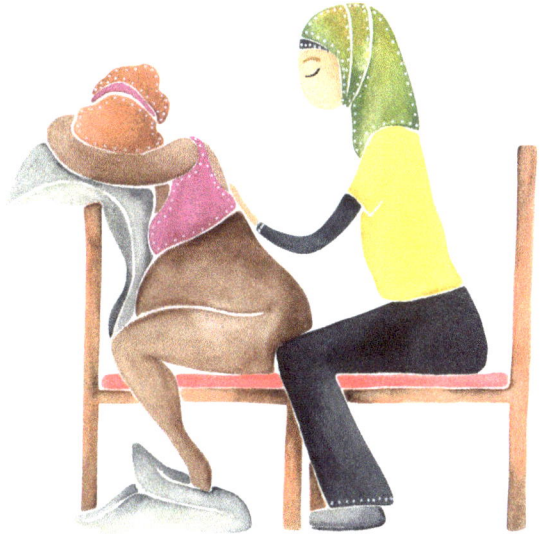

It is easy to rest if pillows or a bean bag supports you.

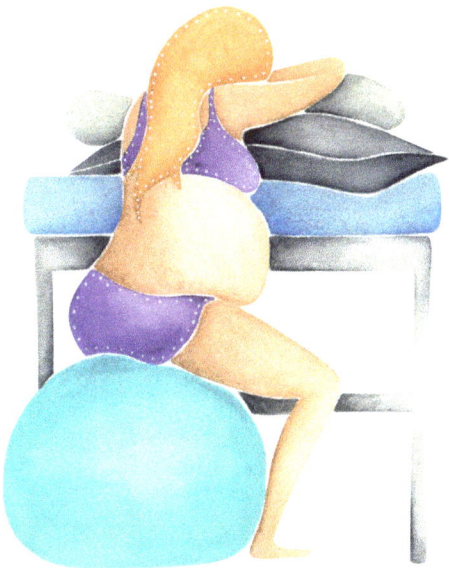

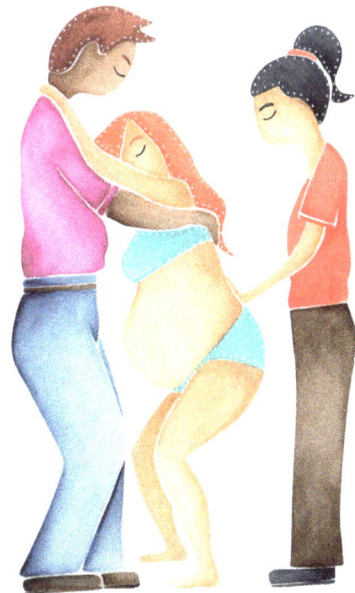

Sitting on a birth ball makes it easy to rock your pelvis.

Positions for labour – using technology

Staying mobile while using technology

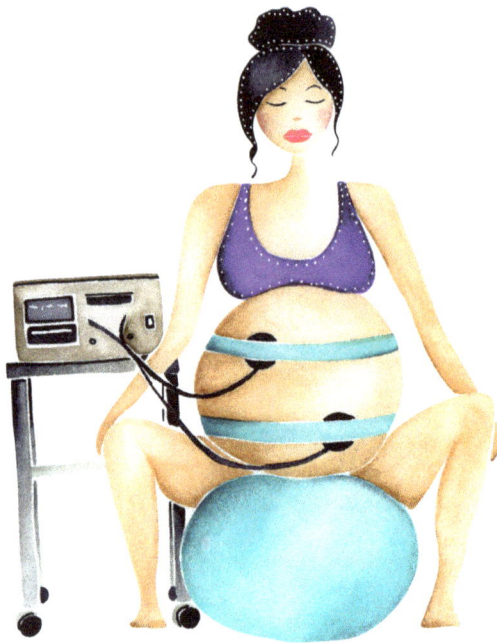

If technology such as an electronic fetal monitor becomes necessary during labour, it is still possible to stay upright and mobile while it is in place. If you use pain medication, some positions may be more challenging to achieve, especially if you have limited use of your legs.

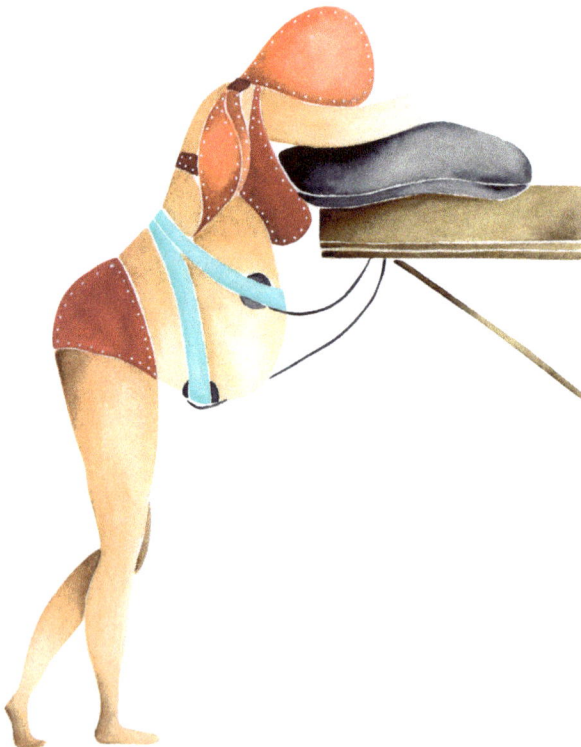

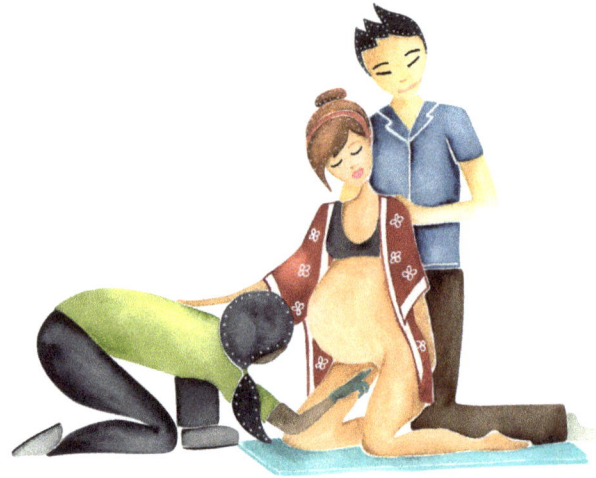

You can ask the midwife to check the dilatation of your cervix when you are in most positions. It is not necessary to lie down for this procedure.

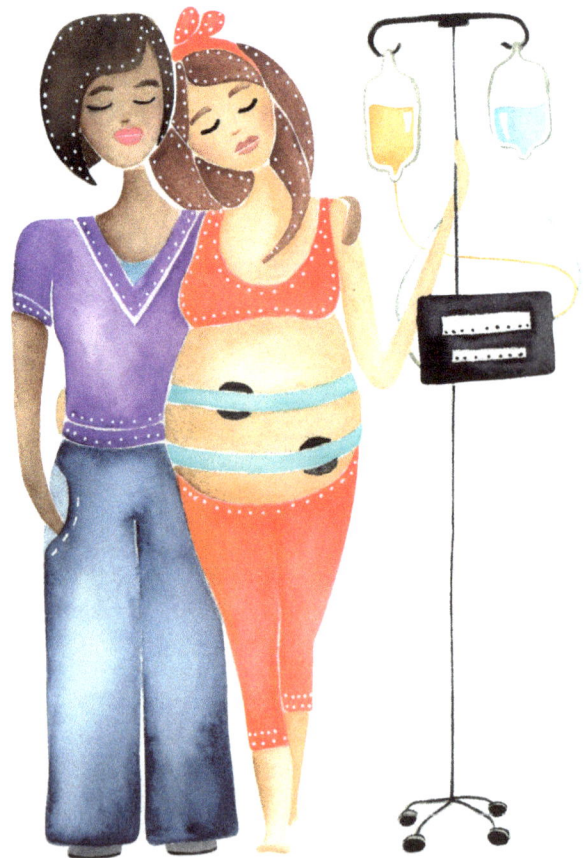

A telemetry unit transmits readings from the electronic fetal monitor to a recording machine. Telemetry removes the need for direct attachment to the monitor with leads and enables greater freedom of movement.

Using peanut balls

A peanut ball is an inflatable peanut shaped birth ball used to help women into active birth positions in labour. They're used to help a baby rotate into an ideal position for birth. This is particularly useful for a woman who chooses an epidural in labour as a peanut ball is used to shorten labour and reduce the caesarean birth rate. Are they successful in doing this? Currently, we don't know, but it's looking promising for lowering the caesarean birth rate. More research is underway.

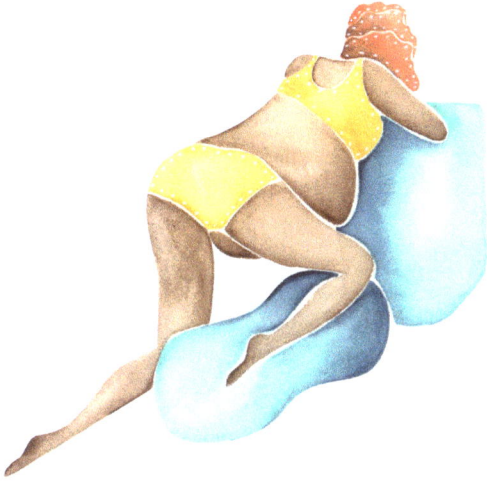

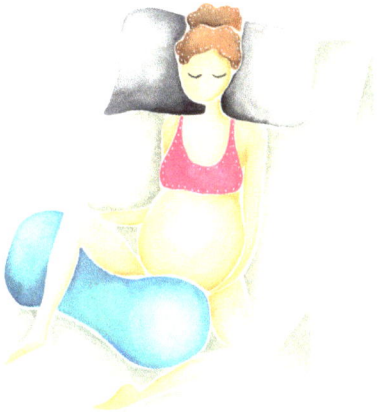

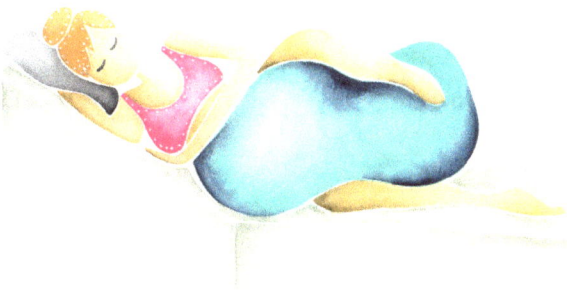

Positions for labour – second stage

In the second stage, you need to brace your body to push effectively. You may need something to grip and may prefer to be upright with your legs planted firmly on a floor mat and with good support from your partner or other helpers. You can also use the furniture as a source of support.

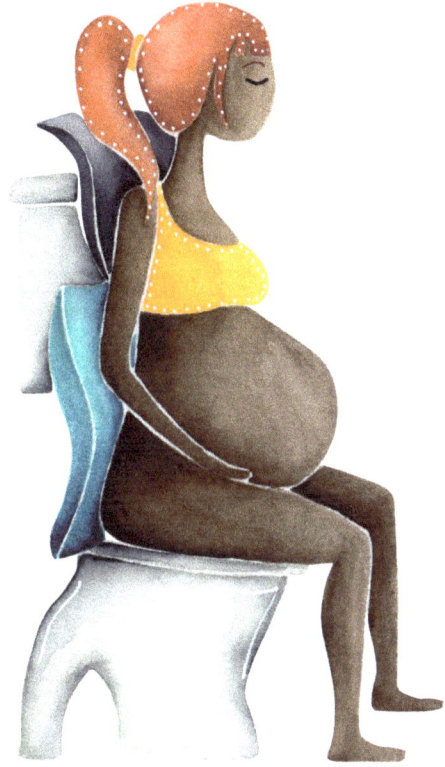

Sitting on the toilet often helps early pushing contractions become more coordinated.

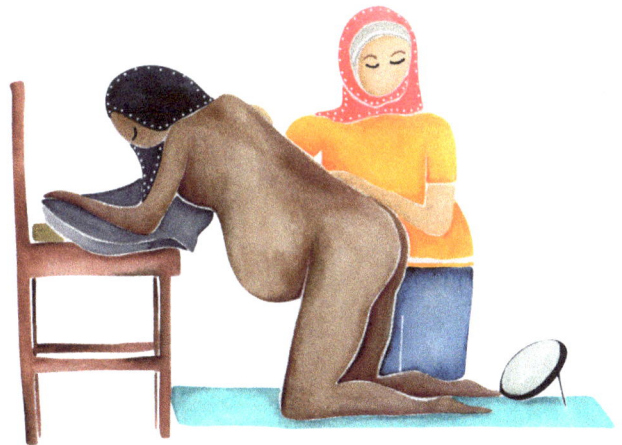

A mirror is helpful to enable the partner, support person or caregivers to see the baby's progress towards birth. Women usually have their eyes tightly closed at this time!

Positions for labour – second stage (continued)

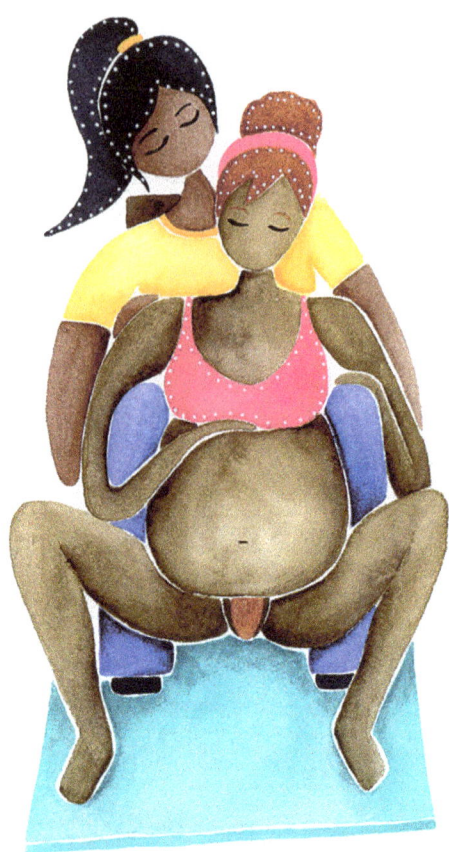

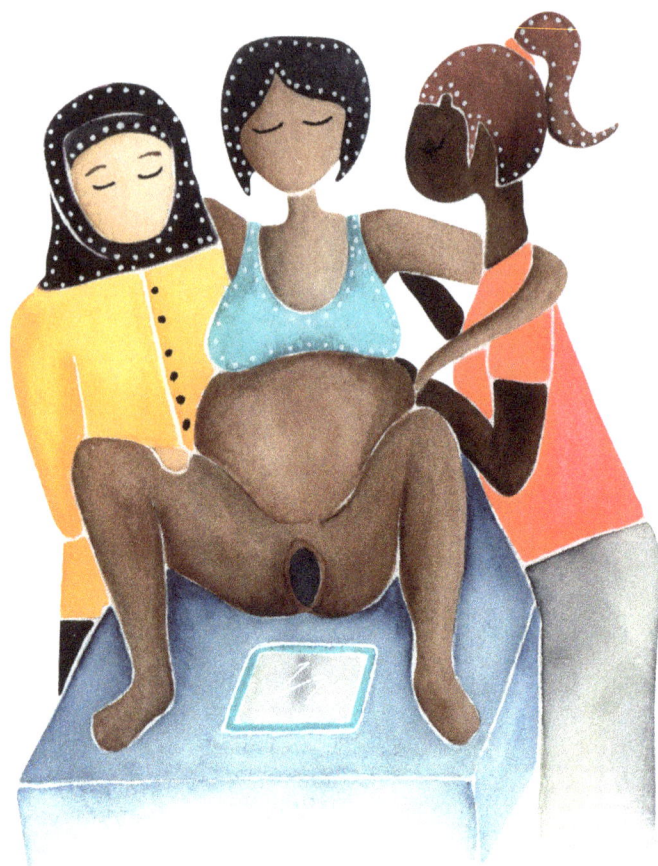

Use a partner or support person to help get into a squatting position.

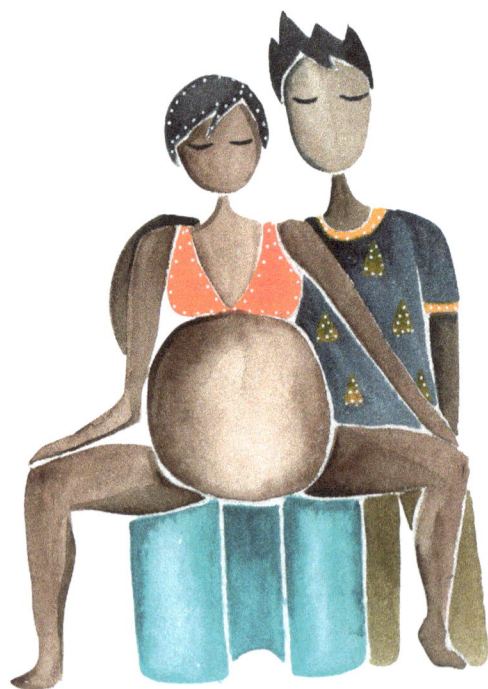

A birth stool can be comfortable support during birth.

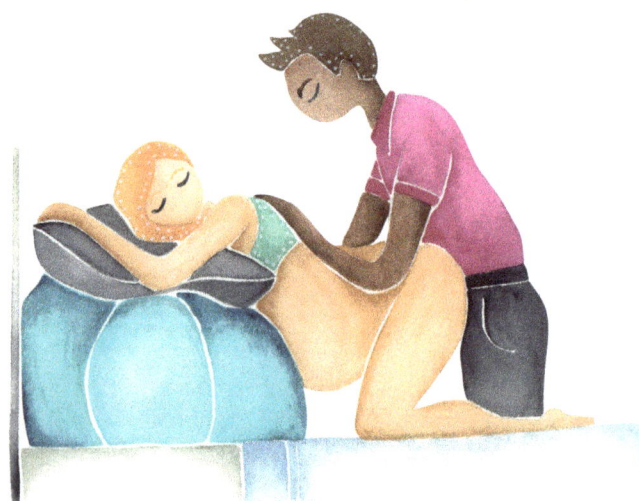

Leaning forward helps reduce the effect of gravity during birth. Forward leaning is helpful if the labour is swift.

Positions for second stage – supported squat

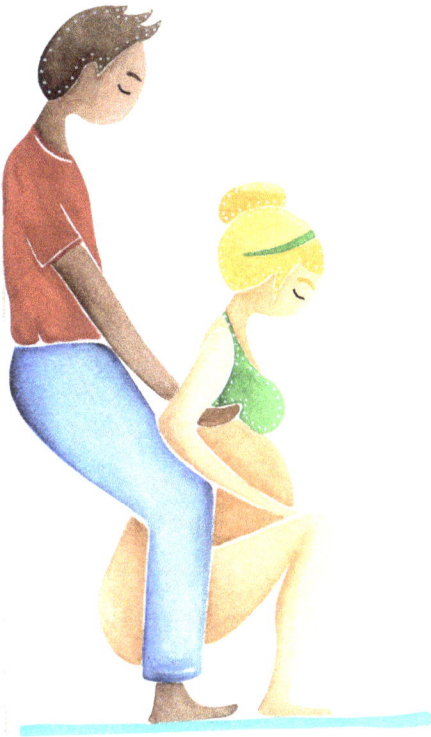

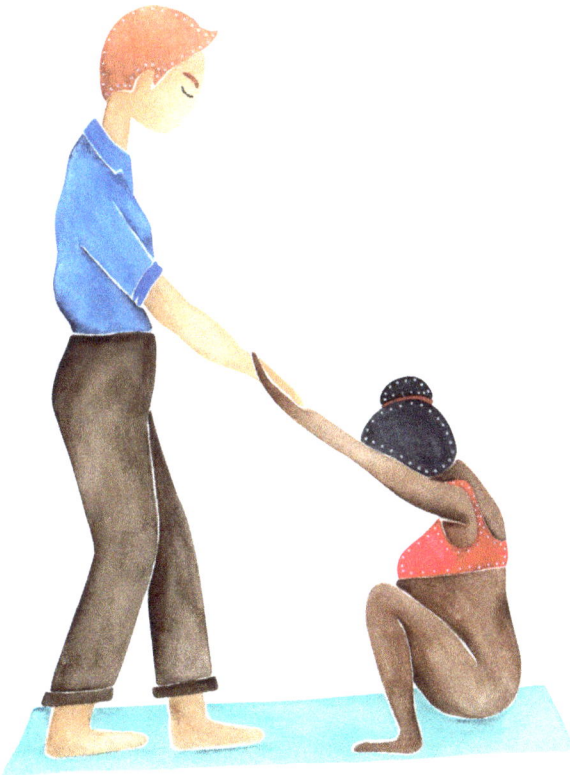

Leaning against a wall makes it easier to support a woman in a deep squat.

Comfort measures for labour and birth

Acupressure

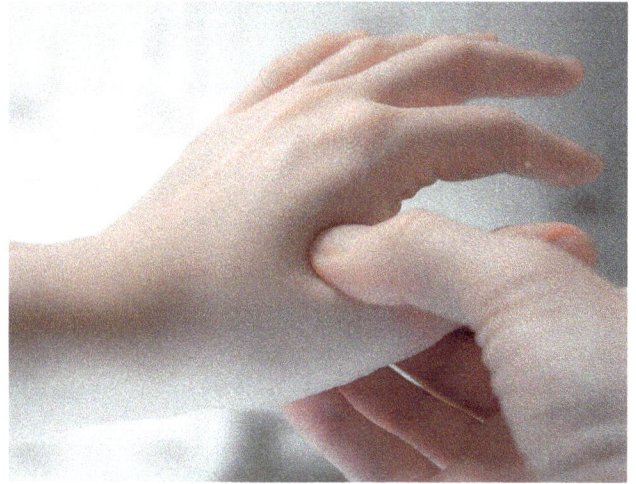

Acupressure comes from acupuncture, but instead of using needles, acupressure uses hands or other tools to apply pressure to acupuncture points on the body by another person. During labour, acupressure may help increase satisfaction with labour, reduce pain or speed up labour. Stimulation of specific points on the body achieves different outcomes. Learn about acupressure from an experienced health professional or refer to *Preparing for Birth: Partners* for an acupressure guide. We need more quality research on acupressure in labour, but current findings are promising.

Heat pack

Hot packs made from wheat or rice are popular. You can heat them in a microwave. It's important to follow manufacturers' instructions on how to warm them. If done incorrectly, they can catch on fire. Alternatively, use gel-filled plastic packs heated in hot water or a microwave. You can use these hot packs in the shower or bath. Apply a hot pack to areas of localised pain.

Massage techniques

Physical touch helps improve the mind-body connection. Massage removes toxic by-products of muscle exertion and eases muscle fatigue. It also reduces muscle tension and can help relieve spontaneous shaking or cramping in labour. Practise massage at least once a week in pregnancy. You may wish to use vegetable oil to make massaging easier.

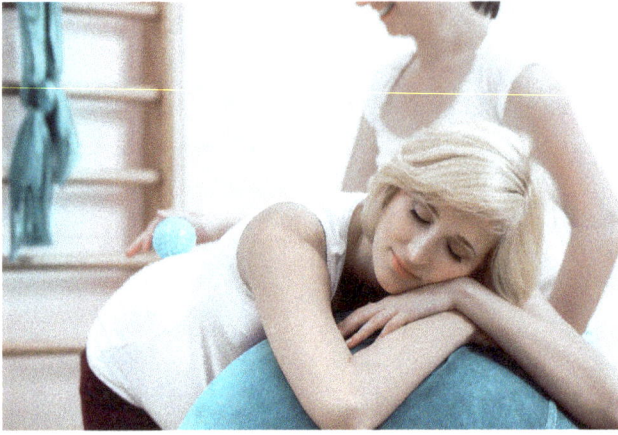

There are many areas where massage can help relieve tension and pain in labour:

- **Sacral massage**: you can do this when you assume various positions. Excellent for back pain
- **Thigh massage**: ideal for cramps, fatigue or shaking in labour
- **Stroking massage**: for tense muscles, especially the back
- **Effleurage**: fingertip massage, good on the abdomen during contractions.

See *Preparing For Birth: Partners* to see how to do different massage techniques during labour.

Touch relaxation

Learn to relax towards your partner's or support person's touch. If they see that you are tense in a particular area, they can place their hands warmly and firmly over the tense part, then gently stroke from the centre of the body out to the periphery so that the tension flows out and away.

Let yourself relax with your partner's or support person's touch so that you are working together as a team. Pay particular attention to areas that commonly hold stress, such as shoulders, back and neck. The face often shows signs of stress during labour, so practise gentle touching on the brow and side of the eyes.

Sterile water injections

Back pain is common in labour, and sterile water injections effectively relieve this back pain for up to 85% of women. A midwife or doctor injects a small amount of sterile water under the skin in two to four locations on the lower back. A woman experiences an intense stinging sensation for around 30 seconds, described like a wasp sting. The immediate relief from back pain from sterile water injections lasts up to two hours.

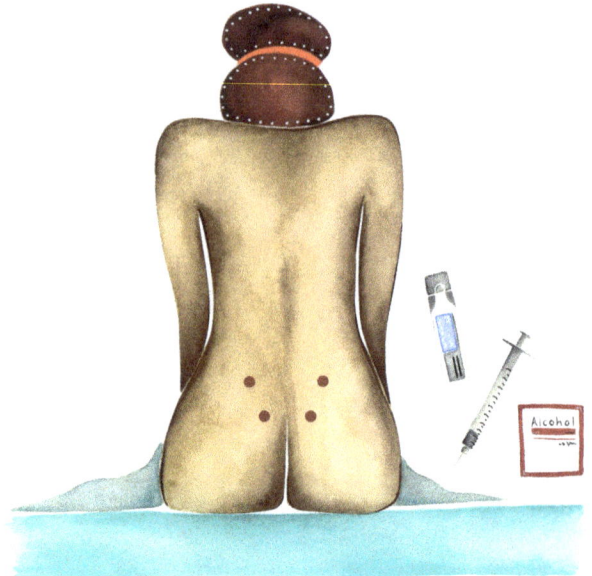

TENS machine

For increasing your comfort without using medication, have you considered TENS during labour? Transcutaneous Electrical Nerve Stimulation (TENS) is one of the many comfort measures available. It's non-invasive and doesn't use medicine – it uses electrical energy. Does it work for reducing pain in labour? There is currently a small amount of research evidence supporting TENS effectiveness. Using TENS during labour is considered safe for you and your baby. Refer to *Preparing for Birth: Partners* – how to apply and use a TENS machine.

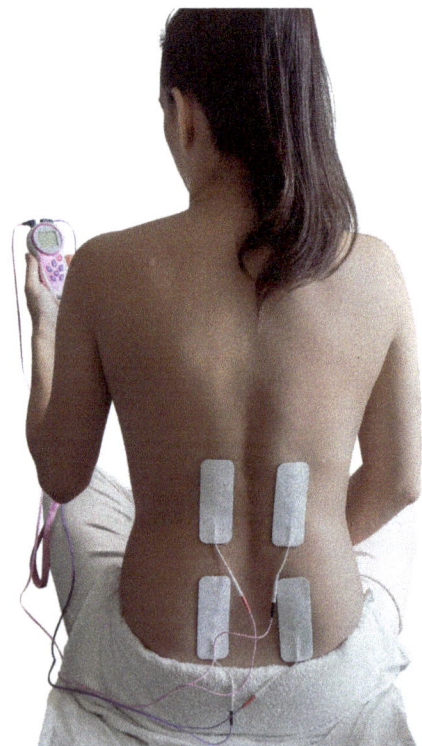

Emergency birth

What should you do if the baby arrives before you reach the hospital or before your midwife arrives?

Emergency birth at home

A tiny proportion of women have a painless first stage of labour or experience mild contractions and are unaware that anything is happening until they feel the urge to push, which is likely to be interpreted as a need to empty the bowel. Usually, the waters will break at this time, which will alert you that this is the baby arriving. Alternatively, occasionally labour can go very fast, and there isn't time to get to the hospital.

Don't panic! This baby is going to arrive at home. If you do happen to be alone, phone your partner or anyone else who is to be with you, summon a neighbour or telephone for an ambulance. Leave your door unlocked.

Go to a convenient place that is warm and quiet – the bathroom is ideal. Get into a comfortable position, with towels beneath you, and allow the baby to be born as slowly as possible – breathe the baby out.

Wipe any mucous from the baby's nose and mouth. The baby will probably cry straight away, but if not, lie the baby on its side on the towels and massage the body firmly towards the head. Flicking the soles of the feet may also stimulate a cry.

It is essential to keep the baby warm – wrap in a towel straight away and wait for the placenta. Put the baby to the breast if possible. There is no need to cut the cord. If the placenta arrives, wrap it in a plastic bag and place it with the baby.

Phone the hospital and tell the midwife what has happened. The ambulance will take you to the hospital. Once there, the midwife or doctor will cut the baby's cord and repair any tears in your perineum.

Giving birth on the way to hospital

Occasionally the first stage of labour progresses so rapidly that you are ready to give birth in the car before reaching the hospital.

Again, don't panic! If there is time, get into the car's back seat where there is more room (you will have to remove your pants). Get into a position such as hands and knees, allowing the baby to be born as slowly as possible.

It helps to keep a couple of clean, old towels in the car to catch the fluids and wrap the baby. Ensure that the baby is breathing and pink and wrap up as warmly as possible before proceeding to the hospital.

There is no need to cut the cord, and if the placenta does appear, wrap it up and keep it with the baby.

Being informed about obstetric interventions

You may find the next section of the book is uncomfortable reading. Some women may feel anxious reading this content. No one wants to think about anything but the perfect birth plan. However, a little bit of knowledge can help you avoid unnecessary interventions in labour. Alternatively, this information may help you make an informed decision should a midwife or doctor recommend an intervention. Knowledge is power.

An obstetric intervention is a procedure carried out by a midwife or doctor that results in intervening in the natural birthing process to assist with the birth of your baby. Obstetric interventions can be life-saving procedures for women and babies. Technological advances, improved surgical techniques and better anaesthetics have ensured that the 20% of women who need this kind of help receive the best possible care.

Discuss any concerns about obstetric interventions with your midwife or doctor. If your pregnancy is uncomplicated, you're healthy and labour starts naturally, you'll most likely not need any interventions.

Cascade of intervention

When the natural process of labour and birth is disturbed, problems can result. Interventions in labour, without a medical indication, can result in the need for more interventions. This phenomenon is known as 'the cascade of intervention' (see the following illustration). Research supports all these links. To read the diagram, start with the intervention and read downwards from that point.

The Cascade of Intervention

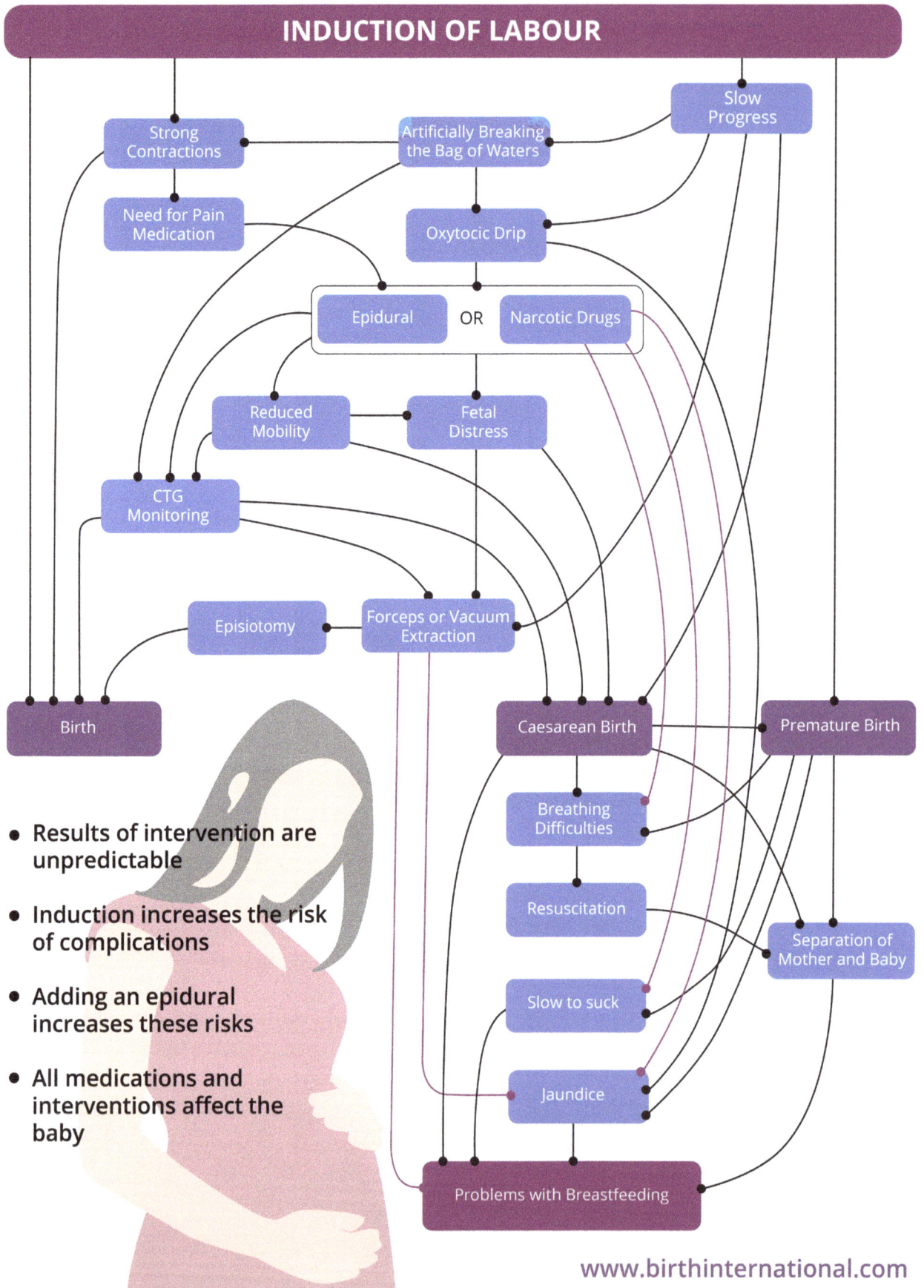

INDUCTION OF LABOUR

Slow Progress

Strong Contractions

Artificially Breaking the Bag of Waters

Need for Pain Medication

Oxytocic Drip

Epidural — OR — Narcotic Drugs

Reduced Mobility

Fetal Distress

CTG Monitoring

Episiotomy

Forceps or Vacuum Extraction

Birth

Caesarean Birth

Premature Birth

Breathing Difficulties

Resuscitation

Separation of Mother and Baby

Slow to suck

Jaundice

Problems with Breastfeeding

- **Results of intervention are unpredictable**
- **Induction increases the risk of complications**
- **Adding an epidural increases these risks**
- **All medications and interventions affect the baby**

www.birthinternational.com

The use of artificial oxytocins in labour

The body produces a natural hormone, oxytocin, which makes the uterus contract during labour. A midwife or doctor may give you synthetic oxytocin (Syntocinon) for three main reasons:

- to start labour artificially (induction). In this case, the procedure often involves rupturing the membranes (see separate entry)
- to speed up labour (augmentation) after labour starts naturally, or if labour slows down, perhaps in response to other interventions (e.g. epidural administration)
- to speed up the delivery of the placenta (active management of the third stage) and control bleeding after the birth.

We will consider each of these possibilities in turn.

Induction using an oxytocin drip

When is it necessary?

If your health or life would be endangered by continuing the pregnancy. For example:

- severe pre-eclampsia (also known as pregnancy-induced hypertension)
- kidney disease
- heart condition
- pre-existing diabetes.

If your baby's health or wellbeing is potentially compromised by remaining in the uterus. For example:

- signs of problems with the placenta not meeting your baby's needs
- membranes ruptured for more than 24 hours with no contractions.

Less clear-cut reasons, such as:

- being overdue
- social reasons
- doctor's or your convenience.

How is it done?

An intravenous (IV) line is attached to a vein in the back of the hand via a needle. A midwife connects the IV bag and tubing to an IV pump. The pump controls a slow release of synthetic oxytocin. The flow rate of synthetic oxytocin increases until contractions are established, lasting one minute and coming every two to three minutes or so.

Effects on you

Advantages:

- usually a reliable method of bringing on the labour if health is at risk
- social reasons: organising the birth when help is available for other children or your partner can be present.

Disadvantages:

- can be a more painful and stressful labour
- increased need for pain medication, such as narcotics or an epidural
- unless the cervix is ready to dilate, the progress will be slow and may lead to a caesarean for 'failure to progress'
- you will be less able to find comfortable positions for labour if immobile in bed. It should be possible to provide a mobile drip stand; however, the drip's attachment into the back of your hand is often inconvenient
- if an epidural is needed or exhaustion results from prolonged, painful labour, there is an increased risk of forceps delivery
- a rare complication is a uterine rupture, even if there is no history of a previous caesarean birth
- increased risk of excessive bleeding after birth (known as postpartum haemorrhage)
- over-riding of the body's natural release of oxytocin. This causes decreased sensitivity to naturally released oxytocin in response to your baby's suckling at the breast, leading to difficulty establishing breastfeeding
- more swelling after the birth, particularly in the legs.

Effects on your baby

Advantages:

- a usually reliable means of bringing on the labour when your baby's health may be at risk
- your baby can be born when specialist attention and facilities are available, for example, paediatrician for 'at-risk' babies.

Disadvantages:

- the increase in the intensity of contractions may cause your baby to become distressed due to reduced oxygen supply. Contractions can be long with little recovery time in between. Stress on your baby increases the need for forceps or caesarean birth in some cases.

- increased likelihood of your baby developing jaundice. Medication used to speed labour or pain relief goes into your baby's system after birth. These medications take time to be eliminated and increase the risk of your baby developing jaundice.
- an assisted birth or large amounts of pain medication, especially narcotic medicines, may cause breathing difficulties and a weak sucking reflex
- early separation of you and your baby if any of these problems are severe
- increased risk of prematurity if your baby's birth occurs before they are due.

Augmentation of labour

When is it necessary?

- if the labour slows down and there is evidence that the prolonged labour is jeopardising your or your baby's wellbeing
- if the labour slows down as a side effect of epidural anaesthesia, synthetic oxytocin helps re-establish the contractions.

How is it done?

The midwife sets up the IV line the same way as for an induction. The only difference with augmentation is that the midwife starts the IV with synthetic oxytocin after contractions commence.

Effects on you

Advantages:

- it makes labour shorter and may reduce maternal exhaustion from prolonged labour
- your baby will be born sooner.

Disadvantages:

- same as 'Induction of labour'.

Active management of the third stage

As your baby is born, a midwife or doctor gives a Syntocinon injection (or sometimes Syntometrine, a mixture of oxytocin and ergometrine) to you. The aim is to speed up the separation of the placenta and hasten its arrival. The recommendation of active management of the third stage occurs if an increased risk of heavy bleeding after the birth exists. If you have no risk factors, active management of the third stage may decrease the risk of experiencing severe blood loss after birth but increases problems following the birth.

When is it necessary?

- previous postpartum haemorrhage
- low haemoglobin levels in the blood (anaemia) could mean a delay in blood clotting
- after induction of labour
- following a forceps or caesarean birth.

How is it done?

- Syntocinon (or Syntometrine) is given by injection into your thigh after birth or into an IV line if available
- the midwife or doctor gently pulls the cord to encourage early separation and delivery of the placenta
- delayed clamping of the umbilical cord is encouraged.

Effects on you

Advantages:

- rapid completion of the third stage of labour
- reduced bleeding immediately after the birth.

Disadvantages:

- excessive pulling on the cord in an attempt to deliver the placenta can cause the cord to break and the need for the manual removal of the placenta in an operating theatre
- high incidence of increased blood pressure, nausea and vomiting if given Syntometrine
- increased need for pain medication for afterbirth pains following birth
- high levels of artificial oxytocin may cause reduced sensitivity to natural levels of oxytocin released in response to sucking by your baby, leading to difficulties with the let-down reflex and establishment of lactation in the first days post-partum
- more women return to the hospital after going home because of increased bleeding.

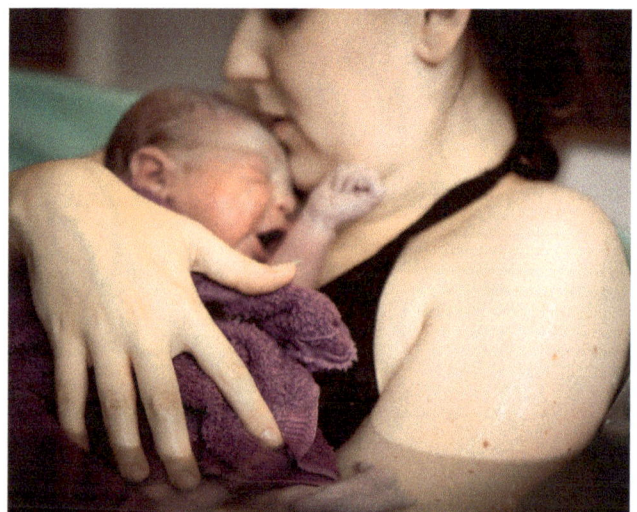

Balloon catheter

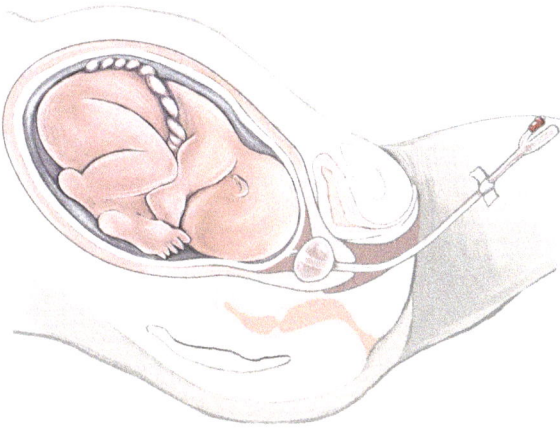

When is it necessary?

- To mechanically ripen your cervix if your cervix isn't ready for going into labour. This is similar in effectiveness to prostaglandin medication in ripening the cervix.

How is it done?

- passing a balloon catheter (thin tube) into the opening of the cervix
- the catheter has a balloon near the tip, which is filled with a saline solution and sits inside the cervix
- the midwife or doctor tapes the end of the catheter to your thigh.
- the pressure from the balloon encourages the cervix to open and for the catheter to fall out
- if after 12 hours it hasn't fallen out, the midwife or doctor will remove the saline solution from the balloon and take out the catheter.

Effects on you

Advantages:

- may stimulate labour without further induction methods
- you can move around freely while it is in place
- depending on the hospital, most women can go home after insertion.

Disadvantages:

- you may find it distressing or painful to have it inserted
- most women need further interventions to get labour going
- increased risk of infection
- higher chance of a caesarean birth when compared to prostaglandins used to ripen the cervix
- potential for an allergic reaction to the catheter
- increase the chance of having issues passing urine
- unplanned rupture of membranes
- may experience vaginal bleeding.

Effects on your baby

Advantages:

- less risk of your baby becoming distressed when compared to prostaglandin
- less admission to the nursery when compared to prostaglandin.

Disadvantages:

- higher chance of abnormal heart rate pattern after insertion
- increased risk of your baby developing an infection.

Prostaglandins

In gel or pessary (like a tampon) form, the hormone placed in the vagina ripens a cervix in women with a cervix not ready for going into labour. It's not safe for women with ruptured membranes or a previous caesarean birth.

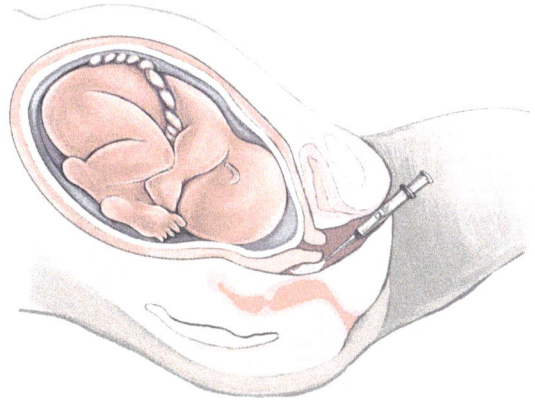

When is it necessary?

- to help soften the cervix in preparation for induction of labour.

How is it done?

- placing the prostaglandins as a gel or pessary in the vagina
- after insertion, you will need to lie down for at least 30 minutes
- one dose may not be enough, and an additional dose may be required
- after insertion, it's usual to stay in hospital for monitoring.

Effects on you

Advantages:

- may initiate more physiologic labour than induction of labour by other means.

Disadvantages:

- over-stimulation of contractions of the uterus
- may not work
- sometimes causes vaginal soreness
- increased risk of fever
- nausea, vomiting and diarrhoea may occur
- potential for an allergic reaction
- increased risk of severe bleeding after birth
- if induction of labour via Syntocinon is also needed, it increases the risk of the uterus rupturing
- most women need more help to go into labour.

Effects on your baby

Advantages:

- may initiate more physiologic labour than induction by other means.

Disadvantages:

- increased risk of your baby becoming distressed
- higher chance of caesarean birth.

Artificial rupture of membranes

A midwife or doctor artificially breaks the membranes surrounding your baby, releasing the amniotic fluid.

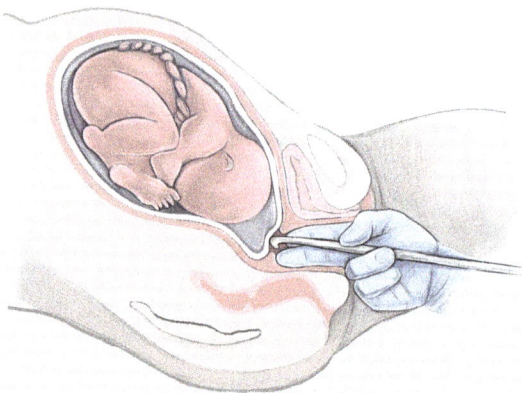

When is it necessary?

- to assist in the induction of labour (usually used in conjunction with oxytocic drugs)
- to speed up labour which has started naturally (augmentation)
- apply a scalp electrode for electronic fetal monitoring.

How is it done?

The midwife or doctor will ask you to lie on your back with your legs open. They pass a plastic instrument with a sharp hook on the end (like a crochet hook) through the cervix. Then they make a small nick in the membranes, and the fluid is allowed to escape.

Effects on you

Advantages:

- may decrease length of labour if used during induction of labour with Syntocinon.

Disadvantages:

- artificial rupture of membranes makes no difference to the length of labour
- the procedure causes discomfort
- the increased intensity of the contractions may cause extra pain and discomfort. Intense contractions may increase the likelihood of using pain-relieving drugs.
- increased risk of infection
- possible increase in the caesarean birth rate.

Effects on your baby

Advantages:

- a usually reliable means of bringing on the labour if used with Syntocinon when your baby's health may be at risk.

Disadvantages:

- the amount of fluid around your baby reduces, leading to an increased risk of compression of the umbilical cord. This compression may reduce blood and oxygen flow to your baby from the placenta and lead to further interventions to help your baby.
- the pain-relieving drugs required by you have side effects on your baby
- risk of bleeding from blood vessels if present in the membrane
- if done incorrectly, your baby may sustain an injury
- increased risk of infection in your baby.

Electronic fetal monitoring

Electronic fetal monitoring is where your baby's heart rate and your contractions are continuously monitored and recorded on a cardiotocograph (CTG) machine. A midwife or doctor interprets the printout from the CTG and assesses if your baby is well or unwell.

When is it necessary?

- if there are complications in labour or risk to your baby
- when there are signs of fetal distress indicating that your baby may be experiencing difficulties during the labour
- after the insertion of an epidural
- during induction of labour to determine the effects of the induction on your baby.

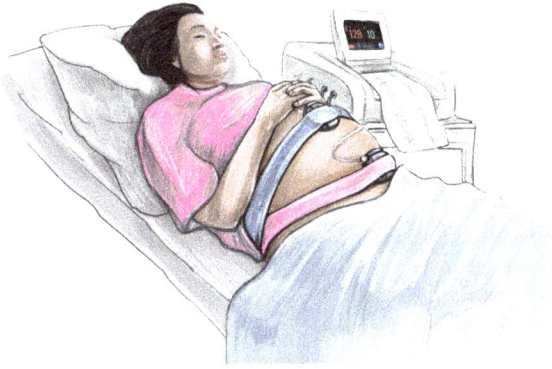

How is it done?

External monitoring uses two large elastic belts positioned around the abdomen. One holds a transducer (a round disc) that emits an ultrasound beam to record your baby's heartbeat; the other belt holds a toco (another round disc) that records the strength and length of the contractions. Both devices are attached by wires to a machine that provides a printout of both readings. Some hospitals will have wireless, waterproof monitoring available.

Internal monitoring provides the same information but via an electrode attached to your baby's scalp (heart rate). Rupture of the membranes is necessary to connect the scalp electrode.

Effects on you

Advantages:

- it can be reassuring to have constant feedback about the condition of your baby
- allows you to visually monitor the labour, which you may be unable to feel if you have an epidural.

Disadvantages:

- you may be restricted to bed and must remain still for the monitor to record well. May limit choices of positions for labour.
- you may find the belts uncomfortable
- transient variations in your baby's heartbeat may cause undue alarm and lead to further interventions, which may later prove unjustified. Research shows considerable disagreement on the interpretation of CTG printouts, even among experts looking at the same graph. This disagreement means there may be inaccuracies in the results recorded.
- because internal monitoring is more accurate, performing rupture of the membranes to allow the application of a scalp electrode may occur. See page 54 for information on artificial rupture of membranes.

- the machine may become the focus of attention rather than you
- research has shown that electronic fetal monitoring is of no benefit in normal labours but significantly increases the chances of a caesarean or forceps delivery.

Effects on your baby
Advantages:

- may enable early detection of potential risks to your baby's health and wellbeing during the labour.

Disadvantages:

- the scalp electrode site may become infected.

> **Recommendations state there is no reason to use electronic fetal monitoring if you and your baby are low-risk.**

Medication for pain in labour

Several medications may be offered to women during labour to ease the pain of labour. Before accepting any drugs, consider their possible effects carefully, just as you would for any drug offered in pregnancy. We've included a list of questions you should ask your caregiver (see BRAIN Decision-Making Tool on page 32). Explore the alternatives before accepting pain medication.

All pain medications cross the placenta and affect your baby, which will vary according to the type of medication and how long it is in your system before your baby is born.

Before birth, you will metabolise and eliminate the drug from your own body and your baby's. After birth, your baby must undertake these processes itself, and this can take some time (days) due to its immature liver and kidneys.

It is impossible to predict how drugs will affect either you or your unborn baby. Everyone has individual tolerances to drugs, with some people finding that they are susceptible while others are not. If you have not had the medication previously, you won't know how it may affect you. It's impossible to understand how your unborn baby will react to exposure to these drugs during labour.

Injections

Several opioid medications may be offered in labour via injection. The choice of opioid medication depends on the current practice of the hospital. Opioid medications are not pain-killing drugs but sedatives and muscle relaxants. They may ease the pain indirectly as you become sedated. Most opioids take about 20 minutes to work and last for two to five hours.

Morphine is becoming widely used and is the drug of preference in many hospitals. It takes effect quickly and is eliminated from your body more rapidly.

Fentanyl is a synthetic narcotic medicine and can be used instead of morphine.

Pethidine is still used by some hospitals. Concerns exist with pethidine when it breaks down. It produces a toxic bi-product more likely to cause breathing problems in babies.

Some women who are concerned about the potential impact of narcotic medication on their newborn baby consider using an epidural for pain relief as an alternative. It is common practice for anaesthetists to mix a narcotic drug (usually Fentanyl) with the anaesthetic agent used in the epidural. Combining these drugs enhances the effectiveness of both medications, enabling less of the individual drugs to be used. However, the longer the epidural is in place, the greater the unborn baby's exposure to the narcotic drug that has been injected, with the potential for the baby to have the similar side effects as narcotic drugs administered through injection or a drip.

When given

This is during the first stage, once labour is established, and generally by injection into your thigh (sometimes via a drip, if one is in place). It's important not to have opiates within two hours of birth due to the potentially harmful effects on your baby. Sometimes opiates are given for pain relief following a caesarean birth.

Effects on you

Advantages:

- sedates
- it has a secondary effect as a muscle relaxant, which may lessen pain and reduce muscle tension, allowing faster dilatation in some women
- may reduce pain.

Disadvantages:

- ineffectual pain reliever for many women
- it affects the ability to make decisions
- creates a 'high', with feelings of floating and light-headedness that makes concentration difficult
- due to sedation, you may find the drowsiness makes it challenging to cope with contractions
- nausea, vomiting and dizziness are all common side effects, especially with pethidine. Anti-nausea medication can reduce these side effects.

- slows labour by decreasing the release of oxytocin
- it depresses your breathing rate, which can reduce the oxygenation of the blood
- opiate drugs cause delayed emptying of the stomach, increasing the risks of aspiration syndrome, a serious complication, if a general anaesthetic becomes necessary
- may cause issues passing urine.

Effects on your baby

Advantages:

- none.

Disadvantages:

- narcotic medication can cross the placenta and depress your baby's respiratory centre. As a result, your baby can have breathing difficulties if born between one and three hours after the injection.
- if your baby has an antidote to counteract the narcotic medication, this gives only temporary relief. Your baby may still suffer breathing difficulties when the antidote wears off after a few hours.
- it may take up to four to five days for your baby to eliminate most of this drug from its system
- separation of you and your baby if these problems are severe
- increased risk of your baby having a low temperature following birth
- difficulties in establishing breastfeeding due to a depressed suckling reflex.

Gas and air

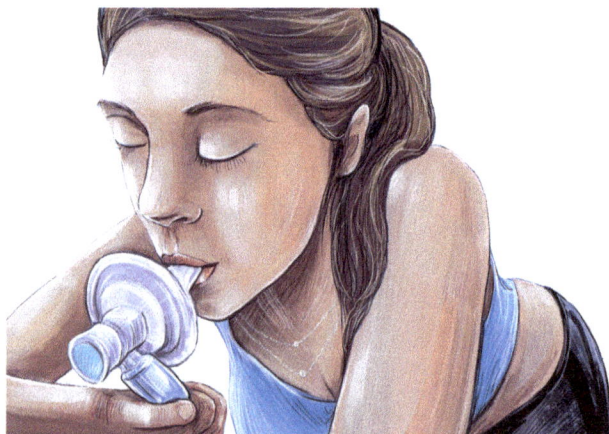

Gas and air combine two gases, nitrous oxide and oxygen, to provide pain relief. Nitrous oxide is sometimes known as laughing gas. Many hospitals use a dispenser allowing the proportions of the mix of gases to be varied within a given range.

Dosage

The dosage ranges from 30% nitrous oxide and 70% oxygen to 70% nitrous oxide and 30% oxygen. Entonox is a fixed proportion of 50% nitrous oxide and 50% oxygen.

Time lag

15 seconds.

Duration

It's only effective while being inhaled and takes a minute to reach its peak effectiveness.

Route administered

It's offered via a mouthpiece, as pictured on the previous page, which you hold. Deep breathing is required to activate the dispensing machine, which sounds like rattling balls. It is essential to start using the mask when a contraction begins to obtain the maximum effect. Removal of the mask or mouthpiece between contractions is important.

When given

When you request pain relief.

Effects on you

Advantages:

- it can be an effective means of reducing pain
- provides a distraction and a focus for attention during labour
- you control the amount you use.

Disadvantages:

- nausea and vomiting can be side effects
- it may make you drowsy and confused
- dizziness is a common side effect
- does not stop pain entirely.

Effects on your baby

Advantages:

- None.

Disadvantages:

- long-term outcomes for your baby are not known.

Epidural anaesthetic

Anaesthetic drugs are administered by injection to relieve pain during labour. An anaesthetist inserts an epidural or spinal anaesthetic. Local anaesthetic, usually combined with another medication, is injected into the epidural space around the spinal cord. An epidural numbs the nerves to help relieve the pain from contractions.

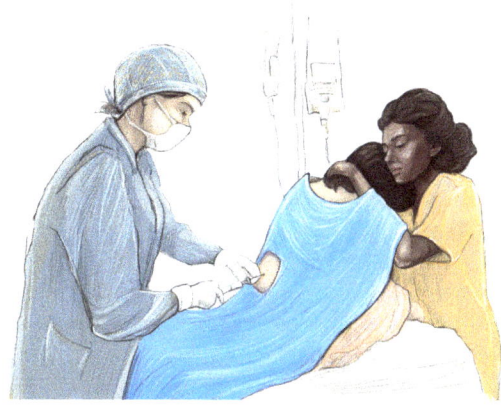

Route administered

A small amount of local anaesthetic and other pain killers are injected into the space around the spinal cord, usually between the third and fourth lumbar vertebrae. After the procedure, regular top-ups of the medication occurs at regular intervals or are delivered continuously through a special pump.

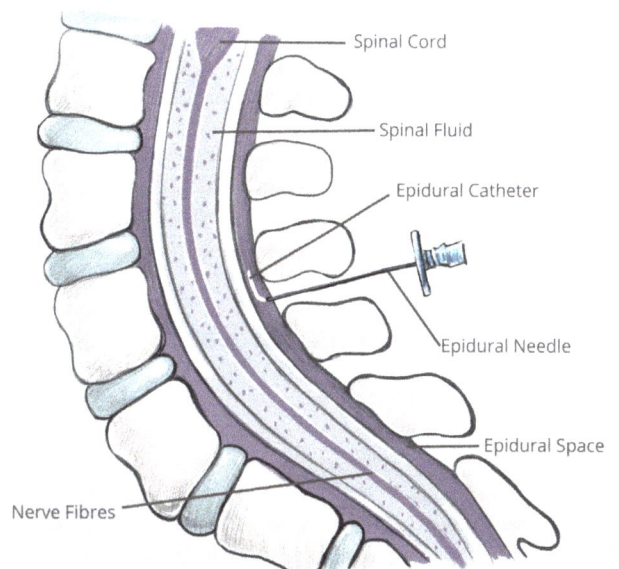

Spinal Cord
Spinal Fluid
Epidural Catheter
Epidural Needle
Epidural Space
Nerve Fibres

Dosage

If the anesthetist uses a full-strength local anaesthetic, then the numbness will be complete. You will be unable to move your lower limbs, due to the anaesthetic effect on the nerves supplying the muscles to your legs. This type of epidural is suitable for caesarean birth.

Most epidurals for pain relief in labour use a mixture of local anaesthetic and other pain killers. This mixture of medication removes the pain of the contractions while not affecting the nerve supply to muscles as much. You should be able to move your legs and sit up while not feeling any pain. This type of epidural enables greater mobility and has fewer side effects. In some hospitals, if the midwife finds you have good strength and mobility, you may be able to stand and move around.

Time lag
Between 5 and 15 minutes following the injection.

Duration
About one to three hours for a single dose. Continuous pain relief for an infusion (continuous release of medication into the epidural tubing).

When given
- for pain relief, usually, once labour is fully established at any time in the first stage
- before a caesarean birth
- to reduce high blood pressure during labour.

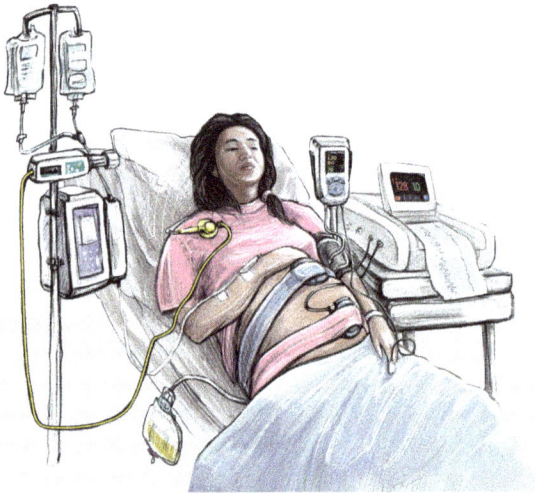

Effects on you
Advantages:

- usually a reliable method of pain relief
- helps to control high blood pressure
- facilitates a forceps delivery if complications are present
- allows you to be conscious during a caesarean birth
- relief from pain may allow greater relaxation and more rapid dilatation
- relieving the pain may increase your positive feelings about labour and birth.

Disadvantages:

- confinement to bed for most women, with a loss of mobility and using upright positions
- in 9 to 21% of cases, the epidural may not work properly, leaving some areas not fully anaesthetised. In many cases, the anesthetist can come back and correct the problem.

- administration of an epidural may slow the labour down, resulting in the need for medication to keep contractions going
- your blood pressure can fall dramatically following an epidural. A midwife or doctor can insert a drip with IV fluids before the epidural insertion to counteract this effect.
- an increased likelihood that your temperature will rise the longer an epidural is in place. This fever can result in further interventions.
- it may be difficult to empty the bladder, and a urinary catheter is frequently necessary for labour
- possible uncontrolled itchiness as a result of the medication
- shivering is experienced by around 35% of women with an epidural
- severe headache following birth occurs in about 1 to 4% of cases due to leaking of spinal fluid
- the anaesthetic relaxes the muscles of the pelvic floor, and, as a result, your baby's head is less likely to rotate, and an assisted birth may be necessary
- you will have a reduced sensation of giving birth to your baby
- tenderness over the area where the anaesthetist inserted the needle is common in the days following birth
- after birth, you may not be able to pass urine, and a catheter is needed
- if your baby is affected by the drugs, you may perceive your baby as 'difficult' and hard to settle, making breastfeeding and nurturing more difficult
- serious complications such as paraplegia are extremely rare.

Effects on your baby
Advantages:

- skin to skin contact with you following a caesarean birth to facilitate early breastfeeding.

Disadvantages:

- your baby will be affected by the drugs used, depending on the length of their exposure before birth. Common reactions include irritability, an inability to settle quickly and a tendency to startle easily.
- should further intervention become necessary, such as an oxytocin drip, forceps, vacuum extraction, or episiotomy, your baby will be affected by these procedures
- any obstetric intervention or complication increases the likelihood of separation of you and your baby in the early postnatal period
- increased problems with breastfeeding following the birth.

Medicalised birth

Episiotomy

An episiotomy is a cut (made with scissors) in the perineal tissues at the time of birth.

When is it necessary?

- if your baby is unwell and needs to be born quickly
- a rigid perineum (the area between the vagina and anus) prevents the baby's birth for an extended time
- if there are signs that a severe tear will occur
- to prevent a severe tear with a forceps birth.

How is it done?

- you will need to lie back so that the midwife or doctor can clearly see the perineum
- an injection of a local anaesthetic to numb the area
- as the head is crowning, a surgical cut, using scissors, from the base of the vagina to the side
- the midwife or doctor uses dissolving stitches to repair the episiotomy.

Effects on you

Advantages:

- an episiotomy may speed up labour by removing the need to wait for tissues and skin to stretch during the second stage
- an episiotomy may prevent a severe tear with a forceps birth.

Disadvantages:

- an episiotomy done before the perineal area has fully stretched will involve cutting much tissue and there will be significant blood loss as a consequence
- episiotomies can tear further, causing a more significant wound
- an episiotomy takes longer to heal and is more painful than a tear, as muscle tissue is involved in an episiotomy. Tears usually involve only skin and superficial tissue and therefore recover faster.
- healing can take months for some women. You may experience sexual difficulties, pain and discomfort until healing is complete.
- having a sore perineum and stitches that require care can interfere with taking care of your baby in the first days post-partum.

Effects on your baby

Advantages:

- it shortens the second stage, and where there is fetal distress, this can be good.

Disadvantages:

- a sore and tender perineum can make it more difficult for you to care for your baby after the birth.

Forceps birth

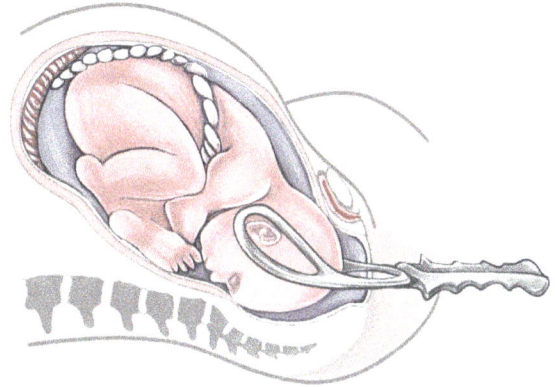

It is a birth assisted with the aid of forceps. Forceps are two blades that lock together and cradle the baby's head as traction (pulling) on the handles helps you birth your baby.

The decision to choose forceps or vacuum will often depend on caregiver preference, training and the clinical situation facing the doctor.

When is it necessary?

Forceps are used only during the second stage, and for these reasons:

- second stage delay, perhaps due to an unfavourable position of your baby or problems pushing due to an epidural
- your baby is distressed and needs to be born quickly
- you are exhausted or have a medical condition that means it would be harmful to push in the second stage.

How is it done?

- your baby must be low in the birth canal
- the doctor empties your bladder using a catheter
- you will be placed in the lithotomy position (on your back with your legs supported in stirrups)
- administration of some form of anaesthetic if an epidural is not already in place
- the forceps blades are inserted one at a time and locked into position around your baby's head
- sometimes the doctor rotates the head into a favourable position
- when you have a contraction, your baby's head is pulled down the birth canal and down onto the perineum

- the doctor often does an episiotomy
- pulling on the forceps, your baby's head is born
- the doctor removes the forceps, and the rest of your baby is born
- after an injection of Syntocinon, the delivery of the placenta occurs
- stitches repair any episiotomy wound or tear.

Effects on you
Advantages:

- when you are exhausted or unable to push, it allows your baby to be born without physical effort.

Disadvantages:

- because it's an assisted birth, you miss the experience of pushing the baby out yourself or feeling your baby emerge
- usually, the doctor performs an episiotomy
- there's usually bruising of internal tissues and additional strain on pelvic floor muscles
- increased risk of excessive bleeding after birth.

Effects on your baby
Advantages:

- where your baby is distressed, a forceps delivery may be life-saving or prevent your baby from becoming hypoxic (oxygen-starved)
- it may be the only way that birth can occur if your baby is malpositioned.

Disadvantages:

- in the hands of an experienced doctor, there should be only minor trauma to your baby. Sometimes there is bruising, tearing of the skin or swelling on your baby's head.
- increased risk of facial nerve palsy, which causes weakness of muscles of the face
- great likelihood of shoulder dystocia (an emergency where your baby's shoulders get stuck at birth)
- higher chance of more extended hospital stay or infection following birth
- rarely, severe injury such as skull fracture or bleeding in the brain.

Ventouse (vacuum extraction)

An alternative to forceps, a ventouse can be used when your baby requires assistance to be born.

When is it necessary?
Same as for forceps birth.

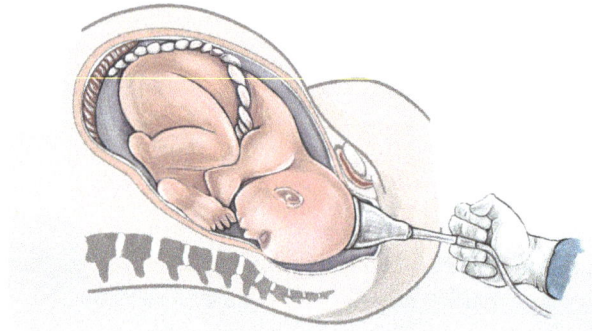

How is it done?
- you will be placed in the lithotomy position (on your back) with your legs in stirrups
- a suction cup is applied to your baby's head and held in place while the suction (generated from a portable suction pump or obtained through the hospital's in-built suction system) draws the skin on the scalp firmly into the cup
- handles attached to the vacuum extractor can turn your baby and gently lift it out
- you must assist by pushing
- once the head is born, the doctor removes the suction cup and your baby is born.

Effects on you
Advantages:

- less likelihood of a severe tear or episiotomy than a forceps birth
- reduced risk of severe bleeding following birth compared to a forceps birth
- less chance of internal trauma compared to a forceps birth
- you can still feel the birth and are involved by assisting with pushing.

Disadvantages:

- the technique may fail due to the repeated inability of the suction cup to stay in place, and either forceps or a caesarean may be necessary.

Effects on your baby
Advantages:

- can facilitate birth if your baby needs to be born quickly
- fewer marks on the head and face compared to forceps. The marks left by the suction cap usually disappear quickly.

Disadvantages:

- not suitable for a premature baby
- a 'chignon' or lump on your baby's head caused by the suction
- the vacuum can injure your baby by causing nerve damage, bleeding on the brain, skull fracture or tearing of the skin. Serious complications occur 1 to 3.8% of the time.

Caesarean birth

Caesarean birth is the delivery of your baby through a surgical incision made in the abdominal wall and the lowest part of the uterus.

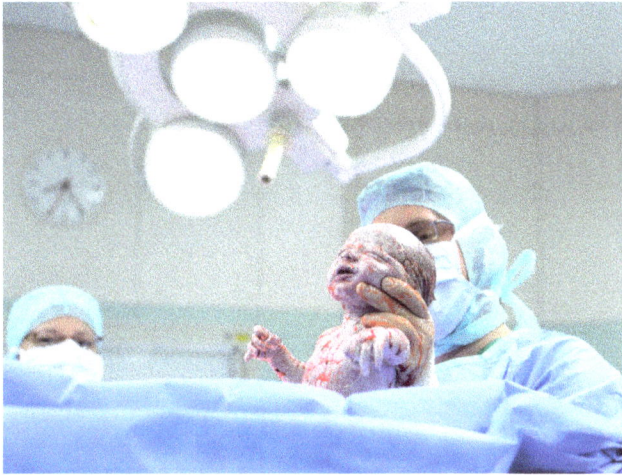

When is it necessary?

- pre-eclampsia (hypertensive disorder)
- fetal distress
- failure to progress in labour
- an unusual position of your baby such as shoulder or brow coming first
- prolapse of the umbilical cord
- antepartum haemorrhage, due to the placenta separating early
- placenta praevia – location of the placenta is over the cervix
- disproportion – your baby is too big to fit through the pelvis
- severe intrauterine growth retardation – your baby is growing poorly
- multiple pregnancy – more than two babies
- fetal abnormality
- distress
- maternal choice.

Caesarean operations are also sometimes suggested for the following conditions, although research supports vaginal births in these cases. Weigh up the risks from the caesarean against any potential gains for your baby.

- breech
- previous caesarean birth
- twins
- history of infertility
- previous neonatal death
- maternal age.

How is it done?

There are two types of caesarean births:

Planned (elective) – if a complication occurs during the pregnancy, which indicates a vaginal birth is risky.

Unplanned (emergency) – if a problem arises during labour.

Types of anaesthesia:

Epidural: the most commonly used anaesthesia unless there is a real emergency. You will be awake during the operation and can see and hold your baby straight away unless your baby's condition requires urgent treatment. With an epidural, you will hear suction noises and feel changing internal pressures and tugging (but no pain) as your baby emerges.

Spinal anaesthetic: similar to an epidural, but faster acting and of shorter duration. It's used as an alternative to an epidural.

General anaesthetic: used if an emergency develops, requiring an immediate operation. You will be completely unconscious.

The specific procedures involved in a caesarean are as follows:

- shaving of the operation site and removal of some pubic hair
- cleaning of the operation site with a cleaning solution
- a catheter is passed into the bladder to keep it empty
- an intravenous drip is inserted into the back of a hand
- a blood pressure cuff is attached to give a continuous reading
- the surgical area is surrounded with sterile drapes, and a drape is erected as a screen, so the operating area is out of your sight
- if the anaesthetic is to be an epidural or spinal, time is taken to ensure that it's working effectively
- if using a general anaesthetic, you will become unconscious very quickly
- when anaesthesia is complete, the doctor makes an incision through the lower abdominal wall, usually on the 'bikini line'

- once through the layers of the abdomen, the doctor cuts open the uterus
- the amniotic fluid is sucked from around the baby after breaking the membranes
- your baby is lifted from within, sometimes using forceps if the head is difficult to get out
- if you are awake, the midwife or doctor may lower the drape so you can see your baby emerging and hear the first cries. It may be possible to hold your baby.
- as your baby is being born, the doctor gives Syntocinon to help the placenta separate. Removal of the placenta is next, and then the wound is stitched.
- following the surgery, you will be taken to the recovery area. Ideally, your baby goes with you for skin-to-skin contact. Alternatively, the midwife takes your baby to the nursery for observation. The partner or support person goes with your baby to make initial contact.

Effects on you
Advantages:

- a caesarean may be necessary to save your life
- the use of epidural or spinal anaesthetics makes it possible for you to be awake and aware during the birth to see and hear your baby being born. Being awake helps facilitates bonding and post-operative recovery.

Disadvantages:

- risks of damage to other internal organs and blood vessels
- risk of excessive bleeding
- risk of infection
- potential side effects of the anaesthetic. See separate entry on epidural.
- lower fertility rates following a caesarean
- as you have been unable to deliver vaginally, you may feel disappointed. You will most likely need comfort and support from those around you to accept this unexpected outcome to your pregnancy.
- separation of you and your baby may be the usual practice after a caesarean, although the time involved may vary according to hospital routine and the health of you and your baby
- increased pain following the birth
- risk of a blood clot developing in legs
- may experience problems in future attempts of vaginal birth
- adhesions or scar tissue can develop following surgery, which can cause ongoing pain or issues with future surgery

- increased risk of complications with the placenta in future pregnancies
- a slightly higher risk of stillbirth in future pregnancies.

Effects on your baby
Advantages:

- a caesarean may be life-saving for your baby
- a caesarean may be less traumatic for your baby than a difficult vaginal delivery, especially if your baby's health is in question.

Disadvantages:

- your baby may be adversely affected by the anaesthetic used
- accidental cutting of your baby during the surgery
- increased risk of your baby having breathing difficulties following a planned caesarean birth
- your baby is less likely to be successfully breastfed
- differences in bacteria that live in a baby's gut compared to a baby born vaginally. These differences may have a life-long impact on the development of the immune system (more research on this is needed).

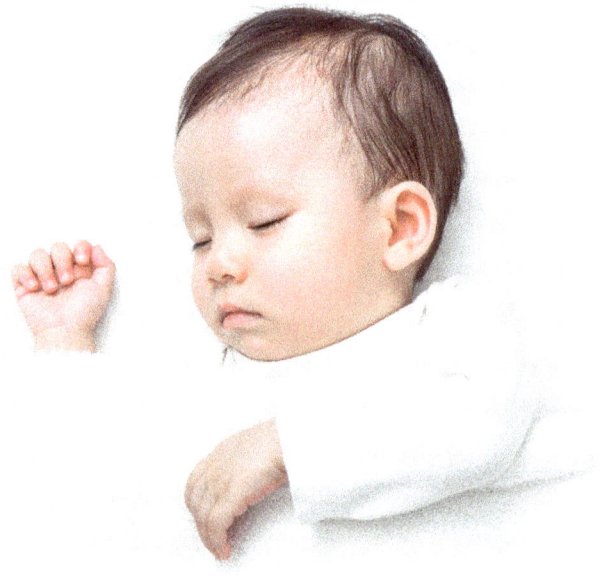

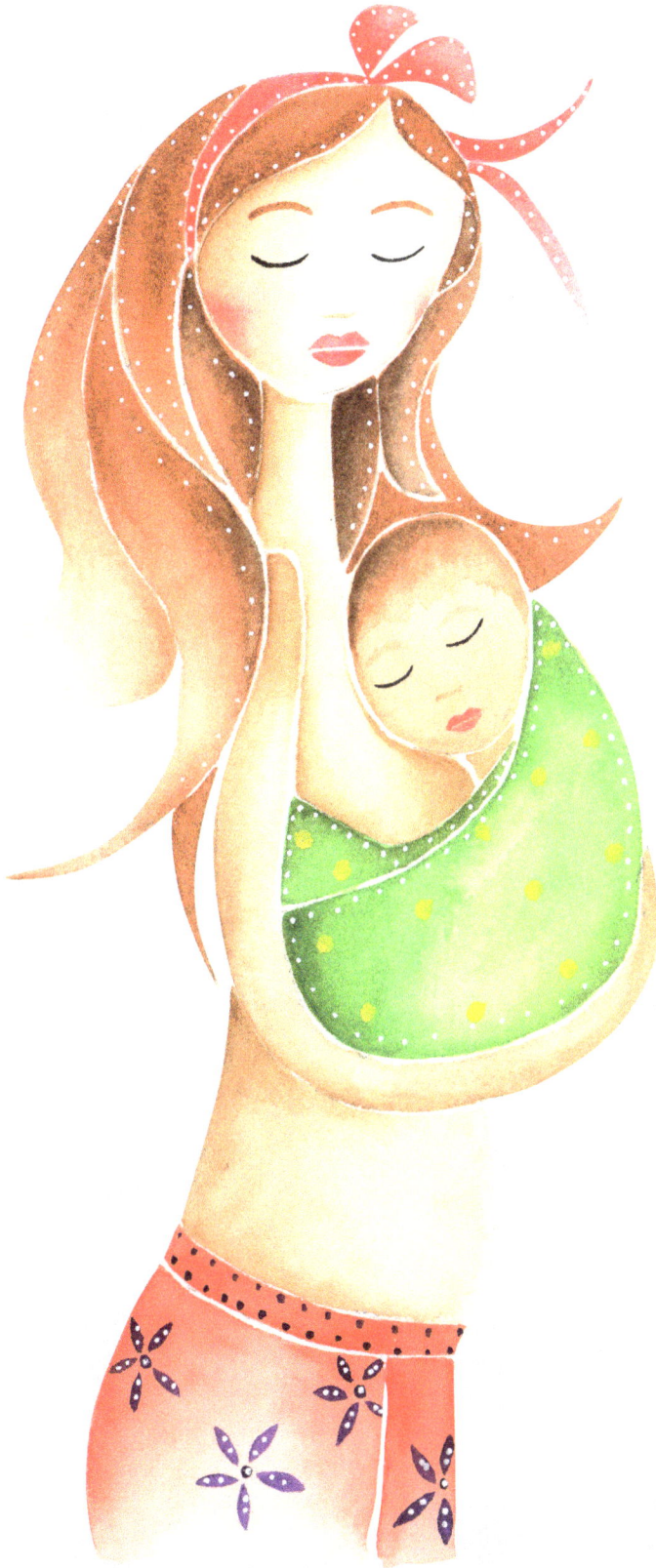

After your baby is born

Your new baby

Your baby will look like an individual right from the start. You may be surprised at their appearance and perhaps puzzled by some of the characteristics most babies show.

Some babies are born with blue bodies and faces. As the baby begins to breathe oxygen from the air, they will quickly turn pink. Sometimes it takes a little longer for the hands and feet to be completely pink, but this is normal.

The baby's head is large in proportion to its body, with a button nose and a receding chin. Their receding chin helps the baby to latch on to the breast. The eyes are usually either blue-grey or brown, and actual eye colour is generally not apparent until they are two years old.

Larger babies are more chubby and have a fat layer underneath the skin, giving them a rounded look. Premature or smaller babies usually have little body fat at birth. The skin may be slightly dry and even flaky in the creases. There may be a vernix layer, a cheesy white substance, which protects the baby's skin while immersed in the amniotic fluid. The vernix can be left on or gently massaged into the skin.

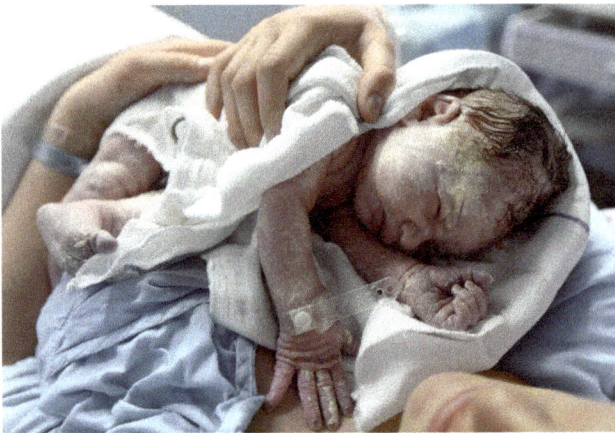

Fingernails are often long and very soft. If the baby keeps scratching its face, trim using special baby nail scissors or nail clippers. You can also use an emery board to file their nails or cover the baby's hands with mittens or socks.

Genitalia appear very large at birth. Boys can have erections right from birth, and girls sometimes menstruate slightly as the baby adjusts to the absence of the mother's hormones. Breasts of both boys and girls may be swollen and secrete fluid at first. Breast swelling is normal and will pass on its own accord in a few weeks.

Most babies will have some degree of moulding of the head at birth due to the pressure as it passes through the pelvis. Moulding usually disappears within 24–48 hours.

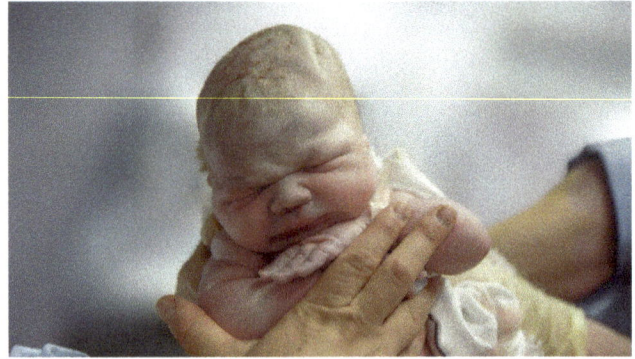

If the mother has not needed medication during the labour, the baby will be alert and wide-eyed. Not all babies cry lustily after birth – some want to look around and take in everything.

Sometimes a baby is covered in fine, soft downy hair. Known as lanugo, this first hair may appear in small patches or cover the baby more extensively. The typical locations of lanugo include shoulders, back, forehead and cheeks. All babies develop lanugo, but most lose it around eight to nine months of pregnancy. However, some babies are born with lanugo. Don't worry; this hair falls out within three to four months of age.

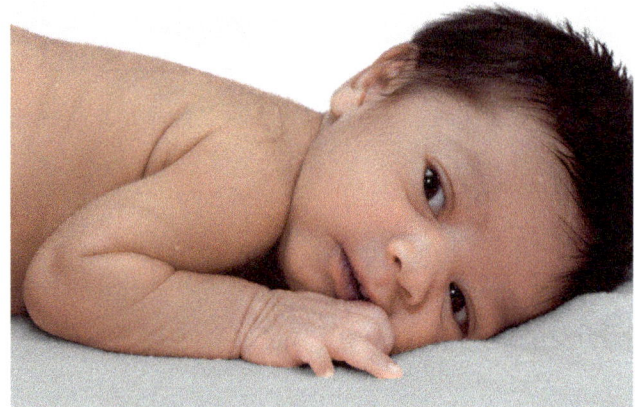

Milia is a common feature in 50% of newborn babies. Seen on the face, generally, on the nose, cheeks and eyelids, milia look like tiny white bumps. Milia disappear without treatment, mostly within a few months. It's important not to squeeze them as they can leave scars.

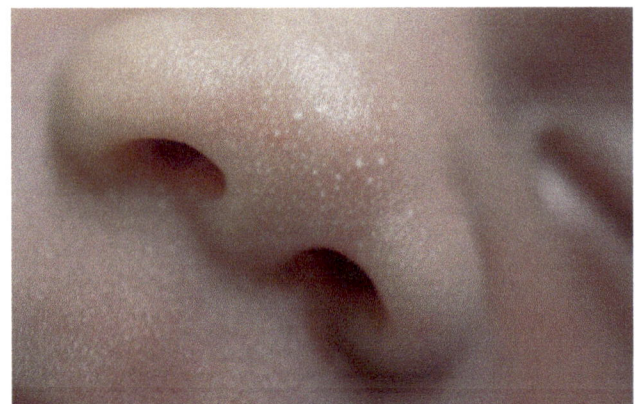

When thinking about newborn babies, we often think of beautiful, flawless newborn skin. The reality may be quite different. Many babies have dry, peeling skin. Don't worry; this usually gets better quickly on its own. Around half of newborn babies develop a red rash called erythema toxicum. We don't know why it occurs, but it's not harmful. Some babies are affected more than others; generally this rash disappears within a couple of days to a couple of weeks.

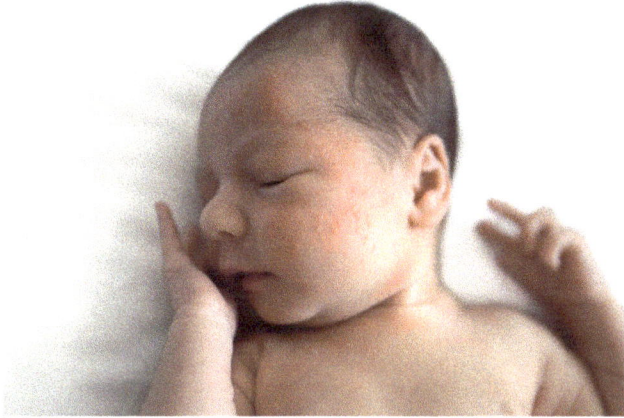

Stork bites are another common newborn feature, appearing on half of all babies born. They are a temporary birthmark, flat and pale pink to red in appearance. Often stork bites are located on the forehead, eyelids, and back of the baby's neck. Immature blood vessels cause them, and they become more visible when the baby cries. Stork bites disappear by three years of age.

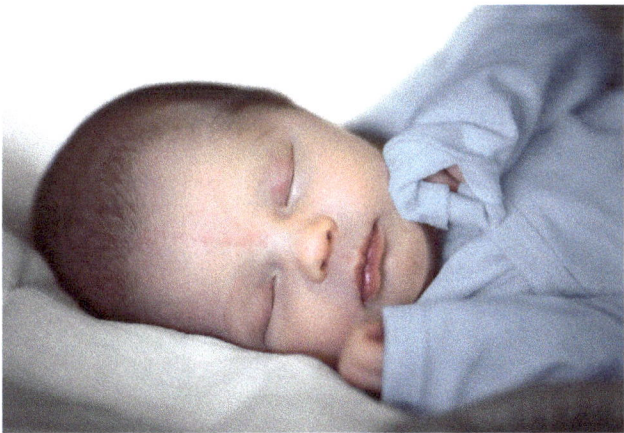

Newborn procedures

Several baby checks are done in the days following birth to ensure that your baby is healthy and progressing well. Midwives or doctors may carry out these checks. Ideally, these tests are in your presence, so you know the result and are able to ask questions. Also, there are various procedures to check the baby's health and detect abnormalities. Find out as much as you can about each test. Talk with your midwife

and doctor about each test to help you make an informed choice about the baby's care.

First examination

Several basic observations are made soon after birth, including recording the baby's appearance, breathing, colour, heartbeat, muscle tone and reflexes. You'll see these observations noted as the APGAR score. The midwife will record the baby's weight, body length and head circumference. A head-to-toe examination will check to ensure the baby is well, doesn't have any abnormalities or a heart murmur.

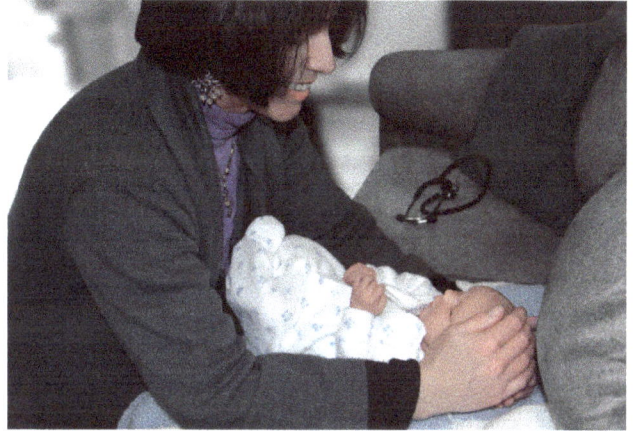

Vitamin K

Vitamin K is essential for the normal clotting of blood. Babies are born with low levels of Vitamin K in their system. Why nature has provided this arrangement is unknown. To protect the baby from the possible hazards of bleeding, especially if the birth was traumatic or premature (with the baby requiring treatments), your baby will be offered an injection of Vitamin K within hours of the birth. The vitamin can also be given orally in three separate doses over four weeks to ensure absorption through the digestive system.

Over time, the baby will make sufficient Vitamin K in its body from the breastmilk to give an adequate level of clotting factor in its blood.

Hepatitis B vaccination

A midwife or nurse will offer a hepatitis B vaccination in Australia just after the baby's birth. The Australian schedule includes four doses; at birth, two months, four months and six months. In countries such as New Zealand and the United Kingdom, the vaccination schedule is three doses from six weeks of age.

Newborn hearing screening

Around 1 to 2 in 1,000 babies born have significant hearing loss. The recommendation is for a hearing test after the baby is 12 hours old to pick up babies with a hearing loss early. The exact timing of newborn hearing screening will depend on the service in your local area. The screener places small earphone cups over the baby's ears and leads to the baby's forehead. They play soft clicking sounds into the baby's ears, and sensors pick up the baby's response to the sound. The hearing screener will let you know the results after the test.

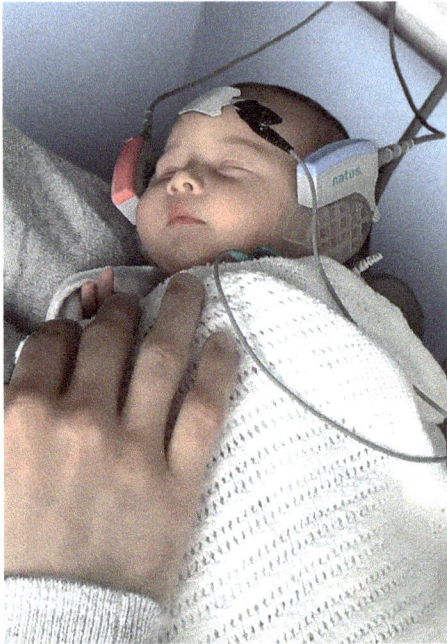

Newborn bloodspot screening

Newborn bloodspot screening programs aim to identify those babies who may have a treatable genetic metabolic disorder. This is a screening test that is not able to diagnose a condition. The screening identifies babies at risk for around 25 different and rare medical conditions that then need further investigation. If you choose not to have the newborn bloodspot screening test, your baby's development may be affected by the time symptoms appear. The most common medical conditions include:

- **Cystic Fibrosis** – a condition that mainly affects the lungs, digestive and reproductive system and stops them from working properly
- **Phenylketonuria (PKU)** – baby is unable to break down a protein found in food, and it builds to toxic levels if consumed
- **Hypothyroidism** – the baby doesn't make enough thyroid hormone
- The newborn bloodspot screening looks for many other **metabolic conditions** that can affect a baby.

The screening test is done by pricking the baby's heel and collecting drops of blood into circles printed on a blotting card.

The card is dried and sent to a laboratory to do the test. The baby needs to be at least 48 hours old before the blood sample is collected. Breastfeeding during the newborn bloodspot screening test helps calm the baby.

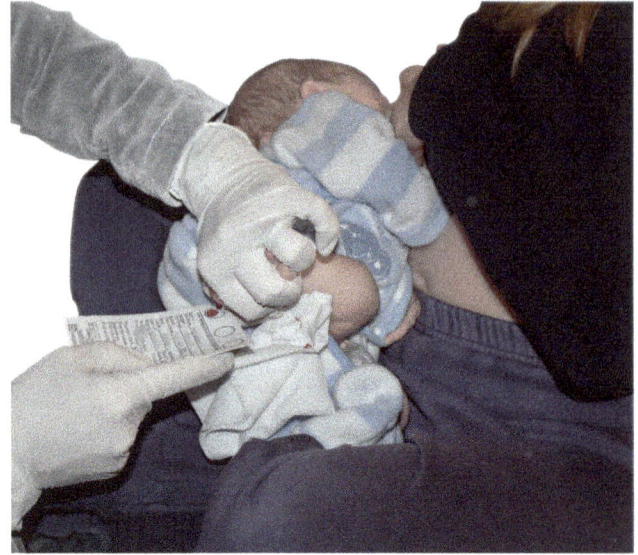

Test for hip dysplasia

Hip dysplasia is where the ball and socket joint of the hip doesn't form properly. The head of the thigh bone is not held tightly in place, making the hip joint loose. Your midwife or doctor will recommend your baby have a test for hip dysplasia. The test involves gentle movement of the baby's hips to see if there is any problem. If any concerns, it will be recommended the baby have an ultrasound scan to check their hip joint. Early treatment ensures good outcomes.

Jaundice

After birth, a baby needs to eliminate extra red blood cells required to carry oxygen before birth. This process causes an increase in bilirubin and results in yellowing of the skin (jaundice). Any drugs passed from the mother to the baby during labour will also need to be eliminated, increasing jaundice levels.

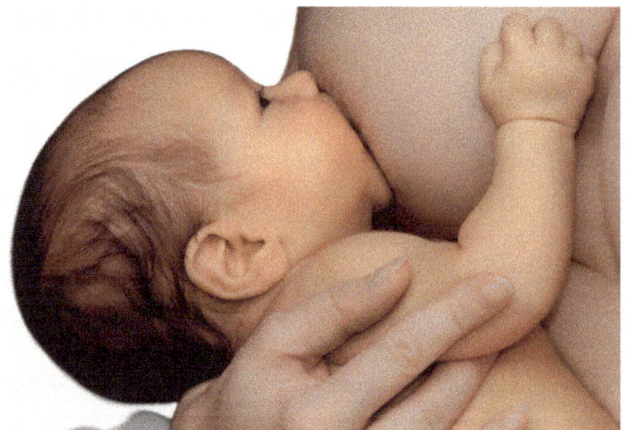

Most babies become a little jaundiced in the first few days, as their bodies eliminate excess bilirubin from their bloodstream. If your baby appears more yellow than expected, a midwife tests the baby's blood test to estimate bilirubin level. It may be necessary to expose the baby to extra light from fluorescent tubes in an incubator to help him or her eliminate the excess bilirubin. This process may take a few hours or days, if severe. While under the lights, a midwife or nurse places a covering over the baby's eyes. Often a baby with jaundice is sleepy.

Continue to feed as often as possible, even though the baby may be sleepy at the breast. The breastmilk will help the baby recover from jaundice.

Circumcision

Circumcision is the surgical removal of the protective skin over the tip of the penis. It's usually done within the first few days after birth with or without anaesthetic. Circumcision when the baby is older is under general anaesthetic.

Unless there is a religious reason or deformity (which makes the passing of urine difficult), doctors agree that circumcision is unnecessary and carries infection risks and risk of poor surgical technique.

It's essential to know that the foreskin adheres to the tip of the penis until the second or third year. Forcible retraction of the foreskin can lead to infection and other complications. When the skin is ready to retract, it will do so, probably as a result of the boy's explorations. In the meantime, general hygiene is all that is required.

Newborn care

Cord care

When your baby is born, their cord will be clamped and cut. Usually, the clamp is left on for at least 24 hours. Over the first few days, the cord stump dries up and darkens in colour. Eventually, the cord stump will fall off within a week or two. As the cord separates, you may see some oozing from around the cord, and it can smell a little. Don't worry as this is a normal part of the healing process. Use water to keep the area clean and then pat the area dry.

Tips on cord care:

- leave the cord alone until it falls off
- don't ever pull on it even if it looks ready to separate
- wash your hands before touching the cord stump

- dry the cord off after bathing by gently patting with a towel or soft cloth
- fold nappies down so that the cord stump isn't covered and allow it to air dry
- don't use any soaps, creams or antiseptic products on the cord stump
- contact your midwife or doctor if you notice redness around the base of the cord or if there is an offensive smell.

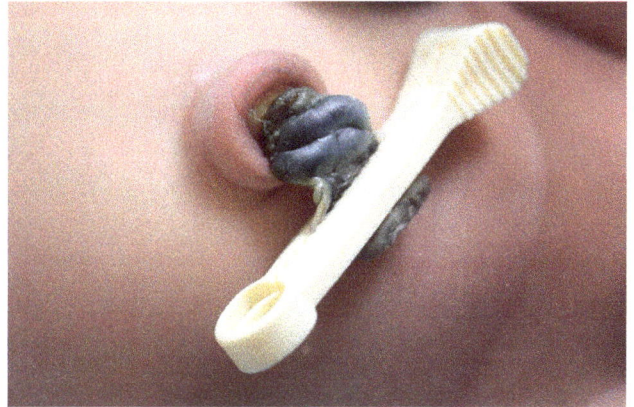

Bathing your baby

If you've never bathed a baby before, a midwife will show you how. A newborn baby only needs to have a bath two or three times a week. If your baby really likes a bath, you can bath daily but be careful not to dry out your baby's skin. Choose skincare products carefully. A newborn baby's skin is very delicate and may not withstand the drying effects of baby skincare products. Gifts of wonderfully scented baby products can be kept for use when your baby is older.

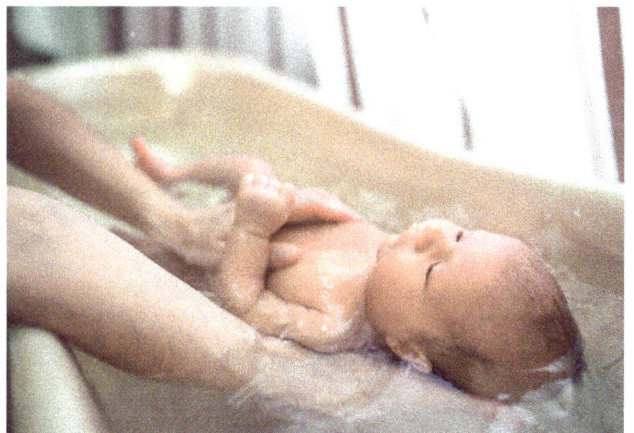

The following tips are useful for bathing your baby:

- Get everything ready for your baby's bath beforehand and have it in easy reach. Don't leave the baby unattended on a change table while you dash to grab something you've forgotten.

- Fill the bath with warm water. The ideal temperature is around 37 to 38 degrees Celsius – check with a thermometer. If you don't have a thermometer, check that the water is comfortably warm (not hot) with your wrist or elbow.
- Wash your baby's face before undressing. Using cotton wool dipped in the warm water with the excess water squeezed out, wipe from the inner corner of the eye to the outer edge of your baby's eye. Repeat using a new piece of cotton wool on the other eye. You can now wash the rest of your baby's face.
- Use your cotton wool, natural sponge or your hand to wash the baby. Washcloths are harsh on a baby's skin.
- Don't use soap – it's best to use just water for the first month of life.
- If necessary, apply a thin layer of barrier cream free from preservatives, colours, perfumes and antiseptics to the nappy area.
- If you decide to use baby skincare products, read the labels carefully.
- Ideally, don't use baby wipes for the first month. After this time, choose ones free from alcohol, perfumes, artificial colours, parabens and phthalates.
- Avoid shampoo for the first year of life.
- Never leave a baby alone in the bath.

Sleep and safe sleep practices

The following tips help you keep your baby safe and help reduce sudden infant death syndrome incidence:

- Put your baby to sleep on their back.
- Have your baby sleep in your room for their first year.
- Make sure your baby's sleep space is safe – they can't get covered with bedding, get trapped or roll out of bed. If using a cot or bassinet, make sure it meets industry standards.
- Use a well-fitting firm mattress in the baby's bassinet or cot.
- Place your baby's feet at the bottom of the cot or bassinet.
- Avoid using cot bumpers, pillows, soft toys or sheepskins in the baby's sleep space.
- Keep your baby's head and face uncovered.
- You should have a smoke-free environment at home.
- Avoid overheating your baby.
- If you choose to co-sleep (bringing your baby in bed with you to sleep), learn about how to reduce the risks of co-sleeping.

Learning to breastfeed

Breastfeeding is the ideal way to continue the close relationship you have formed with your baby during the pregnancy and the perfect source of nourishment adapted to your baby's specific needs. You will find many advantages, from the ease of portability and constant availability to the regular rest periods and extended physical contact that breastfeeding ensures. It is timesaving and cheap and gives protection from disease and infections. Breastfeeding helps the development of a baby's eyesight, speech, mouth and jaw. Breastfeeding also reduces the risk of sudden infant death syndrome.

The first hour after birth (magic hour)

After birth, having the baby skin-to-skin with you is essential. Your baby will be placed on your bare chest and covered with a blanket. Skin-to-skin contact helps your baby adapt to life outside of the uterus, helps initiate breastfeeding and helps you develop a strong, loving relationship with your baby. Missing skin-to-skin contact with your baby should only occur if there is a medical emergency.

Allowing your baby to self latch to your breast is part of the birth process. Nipple stimulation causes your uterus to contract, which helps with separation and the birth of the placenta.

Remarkably, your breasts will help your baby maintain their temperature. Breasts heat up or cool down depending on the baby's needs. A healthy baby who is placed skin-to-skin and left undisturbed will use their instincts to attach to the breast. Avoid interruptions, such as routine weighing of the baby, until after the baby has successful breastfed.

The baby's suckling response is strongest in the first hour, and the nipples are extraordinarily sensitive. This combination means that even if the first breastfeed is not very long or even very successful, the uterus will respond. The baby will have its first sucking efforts rewarded with colostrum – the first breastmilk.

If there is a delay in skin-to-skin contact or breastfeeding, try again as soon as you can.

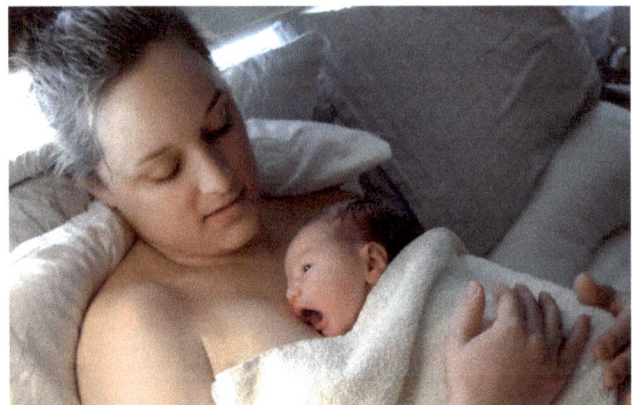

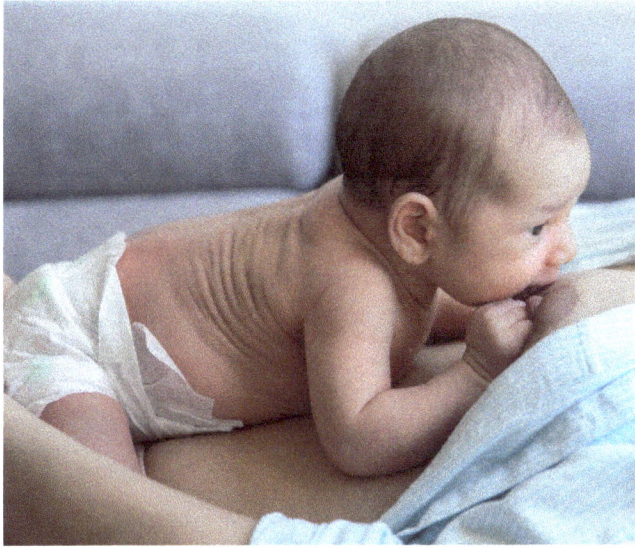

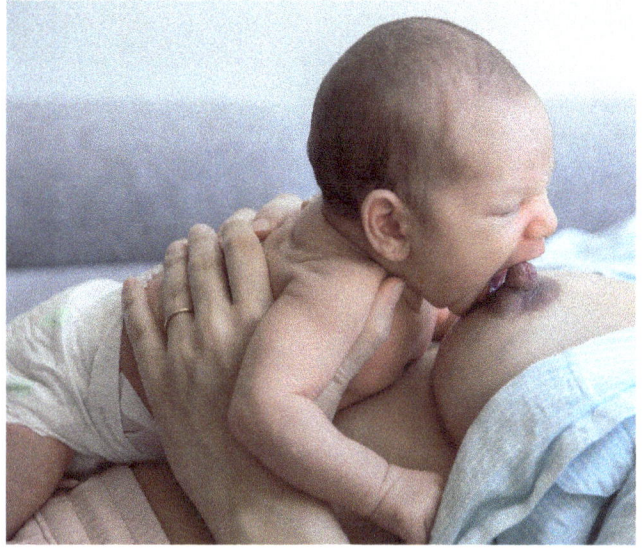

Positioning your baby

After birth, get into a comfortable position using pillows for support if needed. Lean backwards rather than sitting upright. Place your baby between your breasts. Amazingly babies are born with the instinct to breastfeed; you don't need to do anything. When the baby is ready, they will start moving towards the breast, often in a bobbing motion. Support your baby's body as needed in their effort to find the breast.

Once your baby's chin contacts your breast, your baby may latch on without any help. This form of attachment to the breast is known as baby-led attachment and is the ideal way first to breastfeed your baby.

Once breastfeeding is going well, you may choose mother-led attachment. Mother-led attachment is where you put the baby on your breast. Support your baby in a position that you find comfortable, for example, cradle hold, football position or lying down. Support your baby behind their back and shoulders, tucking them in close to you (chest to chest). Do not hold their head. Line up the baby's nose with your nipple. Hold your breast and sweep your nipple from baby's nose to mouth. When your baby opens wide, bring your baby to the breast. Aim your nipple to the roof of the baby's mouth.

You know your baby has a great latch to the breast if:

- baby's chin presses firmly to the underside of your breast (their nose is free for breathing)
- baby's cheeks are rounded
- baby's bottom lip is flared back in an open mouth position
- breastfeeding is comfortable with no rubbing or pinching sensations.

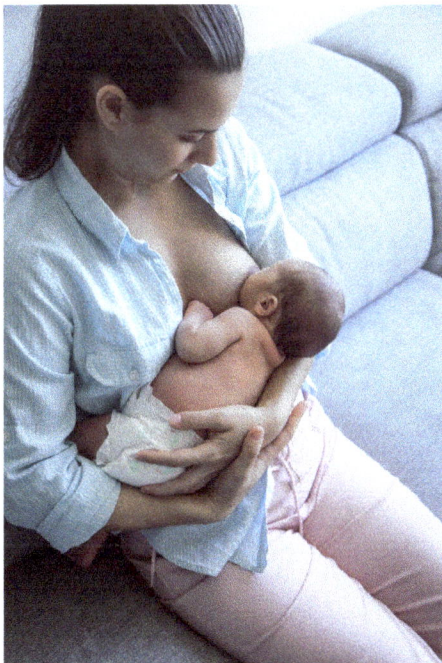

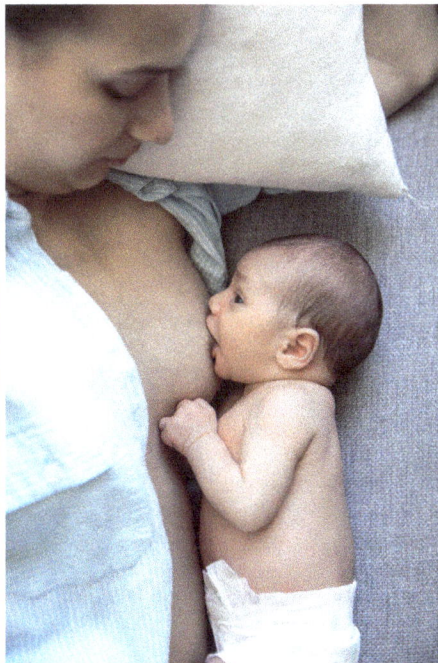

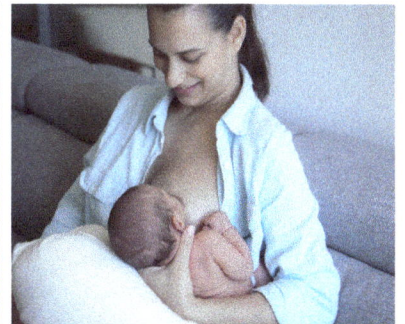

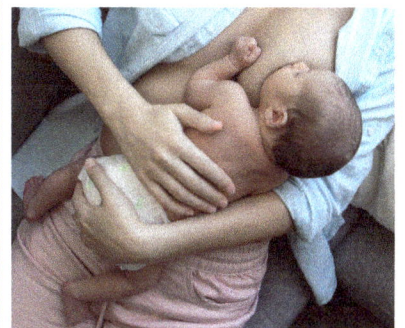

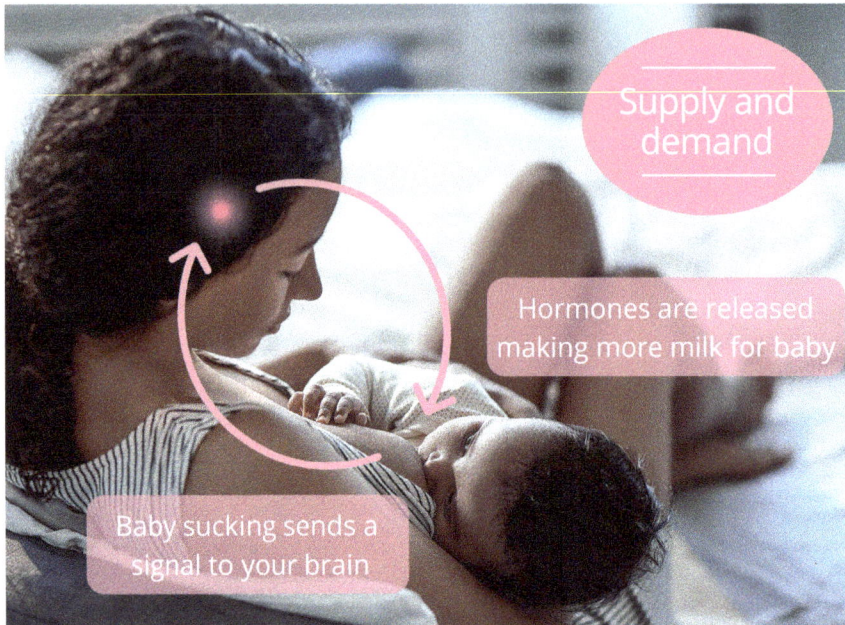

Supply and demand

Hormones are released making more milk for baby

Baby sucking sends a signal to your brain

If you don't get the baby well-positioned, release the suction by putting your finger in the corner of their mouth and try again. There is more than one way to hold the baby when breastfeeding. Experiment to find a comfortable position for you and your baby.

Allow your baby to empty the first breast, then switch over to the second side to finish if your baby is still hungry. Many babies only need one breast per feed. Alternate the breast you start with each time. If your baby is well-positioned, your nipples won't become cracked or sore, apart from initial tenderness as they adjust to breastfeeding.

Breastfeeding is a learning process for you and your baby. You both will learn over time. Many women report challenges in the early days that they overcome with support and correct information. See page 72 for tips in helping overcome early breastfeeding problems. Don't hesitate to ask midwives, breastfeeding counsellors or lactation consultants for help with breastfeeding.

Helpful hints for the early days:

- Health professionals may have different suggestions for breastfeeding. While this can be confusing, listen to all suggestions and take what works for you.
- Breastfeeding is a relationship with your baby – it takes time to develop.
- If you feel vulnerable about breastfeeding in front of others, gently ask visitors to leave. Learning a new skill can be difficult, and it is okay to ask for privacy as you gain confidence with breastfeeding.

How breastfeeding works

Being pregnant prepares your breasts ready for breastfeeding. The placenta produces hormones that stop the full production of breastmilk in pregnancy. After birth, the placenta's hormone levels drop, allowing the breastfeeding hormone prolactin to rise. Two hormones influence breastfeeding. Prolactin is the milk-making hormone. The hormone oxytocin, when released, causes muscle cells in the breast to contract to make the milk flow to the nipple, ready for the baby. Oxytocin causes what is known as the let-down reflex.

When a baby sucks at the breast and removes breastmilk, this sends a signal to their mother's brain to release more hormones to make more milk. This cycle produces more milk for the baby. The more breastmilk the baby drinks, the more breastmilk produced. This process is called supply and demand.

All hospitals should encourage babies to room in with their mothers. Rooming in with their mothers all the time is essential for successful breastfeeding. A baby shows cues when they are ready for feeding, for example, opening their mouths, moving their head side to side (known as rooting) and starting to fuss. Crying is a late sign that a baby is hungry. Breastfeed your baby as soon as they begin to show cues that they are hungry. If a baby is not rooming-in, the mother will miss her baby's cues. As a guide, a newborn baby will breastfeed, on average, 8 to 12 times in 24 hours.

Food or fluids other than breastmilk interferes with establishing breastfeeding. When a baby receives infant formula, it will be less likely to stimulate the breasts to produce more breastmilk. Less breast stimulation equals less breastmilk. Also, avoid bottles, teats and pacifiers when establishing breastfeeding. The use of these items can lead to breastfeeding difficulties.

Do not offer babies any food or fluids other than breastmilk except when there is a medical problem.

Baby Poo and Wee Chart for Breastfed Babies

Day 1 Meconium

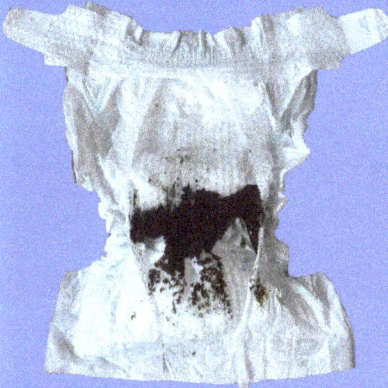

- 1+ wet nappies
- Meconium is baby's first poo. It is black to very dark green. Thick and sticky in consistency.

Day 2 Starting to Change Poo

- 2+ wet nappies
- The meconium is just starting to turn green. You may notice that it's easier to wipe off baby's bottom.

Day 3 Transitional Poo

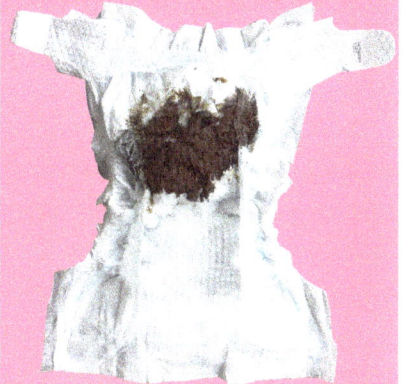

- 3+ wet nappies
- Baby's poo is changing to a green-brown colour. Less sticky today.

Day 4 Green-Yellow Poo

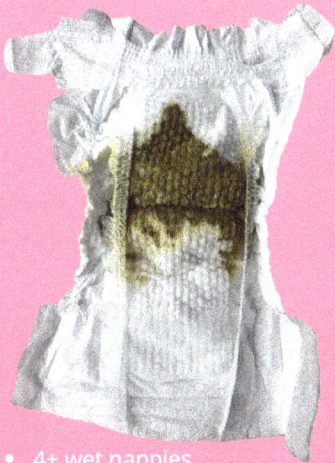

- 4+ wet nappies
- Now baby's poo is a lighter green-yellow colour. The poo can look seedy.

Day 5 Yellow Poo

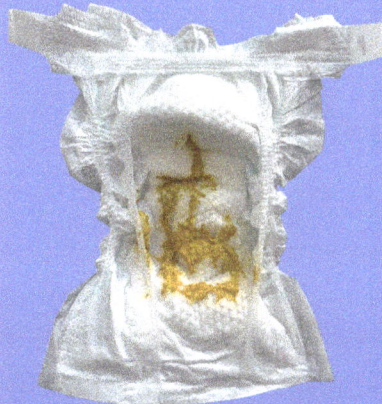

- 5+ wet nappies
- Mustard yellow to yellow poo

Urates Concentrated Urine

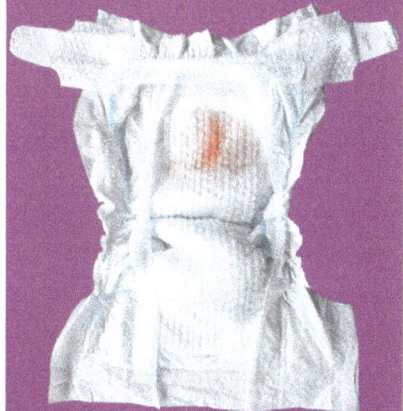

You may notice a pinky-orange colour in the urine in the first three days after birth, known as urates. This is not normal after day three.

Baby's nappies provide you with helpful information

Checking your baby's nappy can help you to know if your baby is feeding well and getting plenty of your breast milk.

What goes in one end will come out the other end. By day five expect a lot of yellow poo. By day six breastfed babies should have at least five soaked wet nappies in 24 hours.

This is a guide only. There is a wide variation between babies.

www.birthinternational.com

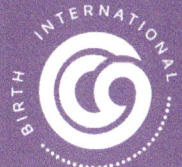

BIRTH INTERNATIONAL

How much breastmilk does my baby need?

When a baby is born, the amount of breastmilk needed per breastfeed varies from baby to baby. In the beginning, the required amount is tiny. However, the amount grows significantly within the baby's first two weeks of life. To give you a rough idea at birth, a baby drinks around 5 to 7mls per feed. By the time a baby is three days old, this amount increases four times to about 22 to 27mls per breastfeed. At ten days of age, the amount has increased more than ten times from the amount needed at birth to 60 to 80mls per feed. A great way to visualise this is to see the size difference between a large marble, ping pong ball and a chicken's egg.

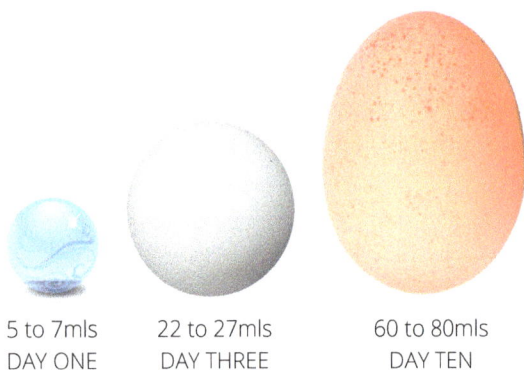

| 5 to 7mls | 22 to 27mls | 60 to 80mls |
| DAY ONE | DAY THREE | DAY TEN |

How to tell if my baby is getting enough breastmilk

One of the easiest ways to tell if your baby is getting enough breastmilk is to check their nappies for wee and poo. For newborn babies, the amount and type of wee and poo changes every day. See the Newborn Nappy Chart as a general guide. The first newborn poo is thick, sticky and black. This poo is called meconium. As the baby drinks more breastmilk, this poo changes from brown to green to yellow. The number of wet nappies increases daily.

Other signs that your baby is getting enough breastmilk include:

- your baby is healthy with good colour, muscle tone and is alert and active when awake
- weight gain after the fifth day following birth
- your baby's satisfaction after breastfeeding (not constantly demanding breastfeeds).

Overcoming early breastfeeding problems

The first step of overcoming any problems is getting high-quality information on breastfeeding while you are pregnant. Knowledge helps you in the days and weeks following birth. Following birth, if you experience breastfeeding problems, seek advice from a knowledgeable midwife, community breastfeeding counsellor or lactation consultant. Don't stay silent; help is available.

Sore nipples

Poor positioning is the leading cause of sore nipples. Check that your baby is positioned correctly (see page 69, positioning your baby). Feed your baby often. The more satisfied your baby is, the gentler they will breastfeed. Before breastfeeding, massage your breasts and apply heat with a heat pack. Try to soften your nipple by expressing some breastmilk before feeding your baby. After breastfeeding, express some breast milk and gently rub it around the nipple. Air dry your nipples. Make sure your bra doesn't stick to your nipples by using a nipple protector. If you still experience problems with sore nipples, seek professional help.

Breast engorgement

Engorgement can occur as the milk comes in around two to three days after birth. Breastmilk changes from yellowish colostrum to blue-white breastmilk. During this transition, extra blood flows to the breasts, and the quantity of milk may increase substantially. You may experience hard, painful breasts. Your baby can find it difficult to latch to the breast. To help your baby, you can hand express a small amount of breastmilk to soften the nipple. Alternatively, you can press down on the area around the nipple towards your chest wall for around two minutes at the sides and two minutes top and bottom (see images below). This technique softens the nipple.

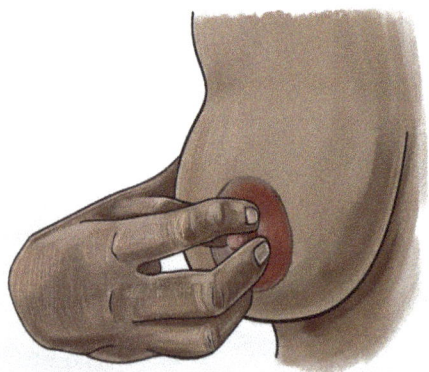

Flower hold

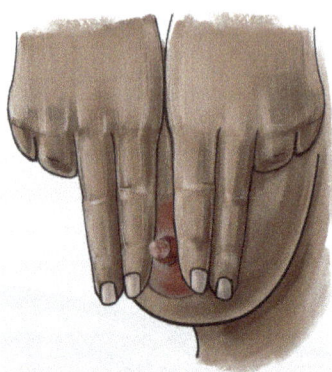

Two-finger hold

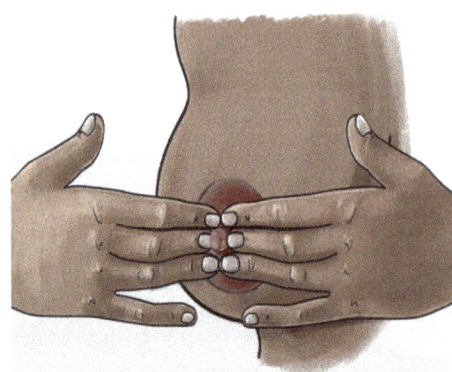

Horizontal finger hold

Apply a warm heat pack to breasts just before breastfeeding to help the milk to flow. Following the breastfeeding, apply a cold pack for comfort. Engorgement settles down as the breasts adjust to the baby's need for breastmilk.

Increasing breast milk supply

The number one reason women stop breastfeeding earlier than planned is that they feel they don't have enough breast-milk for their baby. Check out the section on How to tell if my baby is getting enough breastmilk, on the previous page. Improvement of a low supply of milk supply is achievable by increased feeding. Remember, the more often your baby feeds, the more milk you will make. Here are some tips to improve your breastmilk supply:

- offer extra breastfeeds to your baby – you can repeat these top-up breastfeeds as often as you like
- get as much rest as possible
- eat well
- do relaxation exercises
- skin-to-skin cuddles with your baby
- express breastmilk using a breast pump as often as possible for two to three days. Aim to express every one to two hours. Take a five to six hour break overnight.
- call the breastfeeding support line
- consult a lactation consultant
- speak to a GP or midwife with prescribing rights for advice. Sometimes a midwife or GP will prescribe medication to increase breastmilk supply.

Formula feeding your baby

If you've made an informed decision to feed your baby with infant formula, it's essential to make it safe for your baby. Use standard cow's milk based infant formula, suitable from birth for baby's first 12 months. There is no need to move to step 2 or follow-on infant formula when the baby is six months old. Use specialised infant formulas or ones that are NOT cow's milk based only under medical supervision.

Safety tips

- Make up your baby's feeds when your baby is ready to feed and not in advance. Be sure to discard any infant formula that your baby doesn't drink within an hour of preparing the feed. Bacteria can grow in unused milk.

- It's essential to be safe with preparation, sterilisation and storage.
    - clean and sterilise all equipment used
    - follow the manufacturer's instructions on how to prepare the infant formula
    - follow the manufacturer's instructions on how to store and transport infant formula.
- Hold your baby close with the baby's bottom lower than their head. Hold the bottle at a slight angle.
- Do not prop your baby's bottle with a towel, pillow or other support as this is dangerous for your baby. Always hold your baby in your arms while feeding.
- Serve infant formula at room temperature.
- Using a slow-flow teat, check the flow rate of the teat. The milk should drip out steadily but not too fast.
- Observe your baby's cues, such as stopping sucking or letting go of the teat, for signs that they've had enough milk. Don't force your baby to drink all the milk if they indicate they've had enough. Overfeeding with a bottle can lead to obesity.
- Discard any formula left in a baby's bottle after a feed. Clean the bottle teat and cap thoroughly, removing all milk traces. Infant formula is not a sterile product and can grow harmful bacteria.

Supplies for infant formula feeding

Gather supplies if you've decided to formula feed. You'll need the following:

- One tin of infant formula
- Two to six sterilised bottles, caps, teats and teat covers. Avoid decorations or unusually shaped bottles as these can be hard to clean.

> **If you choose to use infant formula to feed your baby – contact your midwife or early childhood nurse for advice and support.**

Your post-birth recovery

Following the birth of your baby, your body will gradually return to its pre-pregnant state. Your recovery will take several months. In the first few weeks, however, you will notice or need to consider some or all of the following.

Lochia

You will have some bleeding following the birth, and it will be red at first, then turn a reddish-brown, then finally, after about two weeks or so, become a clear discharge. Bleeding immediately after birth is like a heavy period but quickly settles down. The lochia usually disappears after three to four weeks but occasionally continues to six weeks. The initial bleeding will be most noticeable when you breastfeed, as the uterus contracts in response to nipple stimulation. If bleeding persists, mention it to your midwife or doctor at the six-week check-up. If you suddenly bleed very heavily, seek medical advice as soon as possible. Occasionally, women have a haemorrhage caused by some remnants of the placenta or membranes still inside the uterus.

Afterbirth pains

When you breastfeed your baby, the release of oxytocin in response to nipple stimulation causes the uterus to contract. These contractions can be unpleasant in the first few days, especially if this is not your first baby. Afterbirth pains can be challenging to manage. These pains usually become less severe with each passing day, and although a nuisance, they indicate that your uterus is returning to its pre-pregnant size. Applying a hot pack to the area and taking some pain medication in the first few days may help.

Stitches

Recovery from a perineal tear or episiotomy can be uncomfortable or painful. If you have needed stitches in your perineum (the area between your vagina and anus) following the birth, these hints may help ease the discomfort until they have healed:

- If stitches are required, you will be offered a local anaesthetic (if you have not already received this in preparation for an episiotomy). You may find that using nitrous oxide reduces the pain of the anaesthetic injection (see the section on medication for pain in labour).
- Use plain water to clean your perineum. Adding products to the water does not help your healing.
- Keep the area clean by pouring or spraying warm water over the area after using the toilet.
- Change sanitary pads often to reduce the risk of infection.
- Apply an ice pack for the first 48 to 72 hours as needed.
- Do your pelvic floor exercises as soon as you can. These will help improve circulation and speed the healing process.
- The first few times your bowels open, hold a pad against your perineum. This support will help you protect the stitched area and stop the feeling that you may cause damage (which won't happen).

- Lie on your side to feed the baby.
- Warm baths from time to time are soothing.
- Pain medication such as Panadol can help, as can anti-inflammatory medication such as ibuprofen.

Report any swelling, bruising, or anything you may think is even slightly abnormal to the midwives. Stitches dissolve, so they do not need removal. A tear usually heals by four to six weeks but may take longer. If your perineal area is still uncomfortable when you have your six-week check-up, tell your midwife or doctor and seek treatment.

The first few times you have sexual intercourse, use a lubricating jelly. You may also need to experiment with alternative positions for comfort.

Baby blues

Many women feel weepy and emotional between the third and tenth day after birth. Feeling emotional is usually a temporary state and is a passing phase as your body returns to normal hormonal levels and adjusts to having a new baby. Generally, the baby blues last two to three days. With rest, support and understanding, baby blues will pass on their own. Up to 80% of women experience the baby blues. This is the time you need to take extra care of yourself. Don't hesitate to talk to your partner or call an understanding friend or family member. Extra hugs help.

Postnatal depression

Postnatal depression can occur anywhere between one month to one year following birth. Around 15% of women experience postnatal depression. It's important to be aware of the signs of postnatal depression and seek help early. Contact your midwife, doctor or early childhood nurse if you have symptoms for two weeks or more.

Symptoms include:

- low mood
- feeling sad and teary
- feelings of hopelessness or that life is meaningless
- lack of energy
- changes in sleep – not being able to sleep or wanting to sleep all the time
- feelings of inadequacy
- inability to cope
- loss of appetite or overeating
- difficulties with concentration
- feeling anxious or panicky
- feeling irritable or angry towards the baby or family members.

After birth

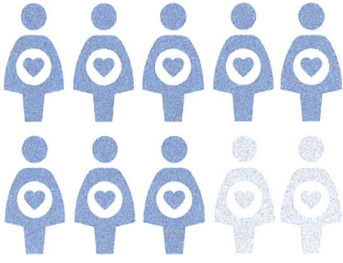

Up to
80%
of women

Experience
baby blues

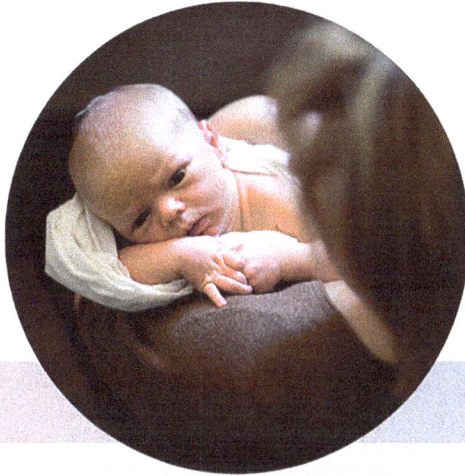

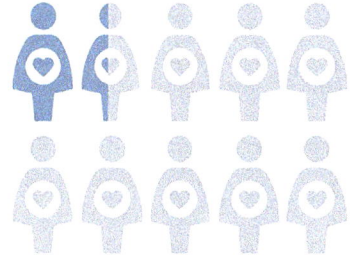

Around
15%
of women

Experience
postnatal depression

Fatigue

The most common problem facing every new mother is fatigue. Broken sleep, natural anxiety about baby care and wellbeing, and hurried or skimpy meals contribute to tiredness. Tiredness can affect your enjoyment of your baby and interfere with your relationship with your partner.

In the first few weeks, make time each day to rest and compensate for lost sleep at night. Having a daily nap helps reduce fatigue. Feed the baby lying down and doze afterwards for as long as you can. Try to make night feeds quicker by avoiding nappy changing (and disturbing or waking the baby) unless necessary. Try to limit visitors to times when you have extra help available so your helper can cater to your visitor's needs.

Make sure that your diet is adequate. Cook up extra servings whenever possible, so you have ready-made meals for busy times or lunches. Eat nourishing snacks, such as boiled eggs, cheese sticks, fruit, cold cooked chicken, wholemeal bread. An afternoon snack containing wholegrain with some fruit and a glass of milk will provide energy for the hectic time in the evening when most babies are awake and sometimes irritable.

Routines

It's impossible to have any kind of routine in the first few months with a new baby. Gradually a pattern will emerge, but it will take perhaps as long as 12 months for regular sleep and feed times to develop. Meanwhile, take cues from the baby and respond to the baby's needs rather than expect your baby to conform to your desired routines. When your baby is happy, everyone else will be satisfied too. It helps to reassess priorities in housework to eliminate unnecessary chores. It is more worthwhile to spend time with your baby either playing or cuddling than having a spotless house, and you'll find that eventually, the baby will need less attention, and you can give the house some extra care.

Getting help

If you have a baby who cries a lot, is hard to settle or sleeps very little, it's helpful to call on others for support or advice. Your local early childhood nurse or health visitor will have names of local mothers' groups, breastfeeding support groups or playgroups.

Talking to other mothers is a big help and very reassuring. Many good books will assist with suggestions.

Contraception

You need to consider using contraception as soon as you want to resume having sex. Many women want to delay this until the six-week check-up, but you need not wait that long if any stitches have healed and you feel ready. If you have had a caesarean, you will want to wait until the scar's healing is complete.

If you are breastfeeding, you will find that vaginal dryness may be a problem at first due to your changed hormone levels and a low oestrogen level. Use some lubrication and take it very gently the first few times.

If you are not breastfeeding, you will have your first period usually four to six weeks after the baby is born. If you are breastfeeding, ovulation is likely to be delayed for some time, but as soon as your baby starts sleeping longer at night or takes food other than breastmilk, then you are more likely to resume ovulation. To be safe, you need to decide when the baby is born to use contraception, even though a breastfeeding mother may have months before ovulation begins again.

The non-breastfeeding mother can use any of the contraceptives available. For the breastfeeding mother, the range of contraceptives is more limited.

Discuss contraception with your midwife or doctor at the six-week check-up or with a women's health counsellor soon after the birth. If you are breastfeeding, you need to consider yourself and the baby when you make your choice. If the method you choose does not suit you or has unpleasant side effects, change to another method. See guidance for your decision if necessary.

Lactational Amenorrhoea Method (LAM)

LAM, if followed carefully, can offer 98% protection in the first six months after birth, providing your periods have not returned and your baby is fully breastfed (no other food or fluids). It is essential to breastfeed exclusively (no supplementary formula, water or solid food) and at frequent intervals both day and night (no gap of more than six hours).

Mini pill

The mini-pill contains progestogen that thickens the cervical mucous, making implantation of a fertilised egg difficult. Sometimes it can prevent the ovaries from releasing an egg. It must be taken at the same time each day. The mini pill may not work if you vomit, have severe diarrhoea or take it more than three hours after it was due. Some medications may also stop it from working. The low amount of hormone is thought not to impact the breastmilk supply or the baby.

IUD (Intra-Uterine Device)

An IUD is a small T-shaped device that has a nylon string on the end. A specially trained doctor or nurse inserts it inside the uterus. Most commonly an IUD is inserted after the six-week check-up. There are two types: copper or hormonal (progesterone). An IUD lasts five to 10 years. An IUD's presence decreases the chance of implantation of a fertilised egg. The hormonal IUD reduces ovulation and thickens cervical mucus. It is considered safe with breastfeeding and can be removed at any time.

Contraceptive injection (Depo)

Contraceptive injections are a long-acting, reversible injection of progesterone that can be given soon after birth. Each injection lasts three months with the high levels of progesterone blocking ovulation and therefore conception. A secondary effect is thickening of the cervical mucous which also reduces the chance of pregnancy. While some women report irregular bleeding, weight gain and abdominal cramping, it appears to be safe for the babies of breastfeeding mothers.

Contraceptive implants

Contraceptive implants offer the most effective long-term contraception method. A flexible rod containing a progestin hormone is inserted under the skin. The rod slowly releases the hormone that blocks or reduces ovulation for up to three years. Removal of the implant reverses the effects within days and normal ovulation will resume.

The use of implants does not appear to have any impact on breastfeeding success or on the baby's growth and development.

Diaphragms

Diaphragms need to be refitted after having a baby and also if there is much change in body weight in the following months. Do not use a diaphragm until your baby is at least six weeks old. They are 92 to 96% effective if used correctly and with a spermicide. If you have not used one before, make sure you are shown how to insert it when you are fitted.

Condoms

Condoms are a simple alternative. Effectiveness of condoms ranges from 95 to 99% if used correctly. You may need lubrication if the vagina is dry.

Natural family planning

Natural family planning methods are difficult to learn while you are breastfeeding, and periods are absent or irregular. To be successful, you must understand the technique from a fully qualified counsellor, who will teach you the signs of fertility and show you how to record them.

Sterilisation

Sterilisation by tubal ligation, vasectomy or the use of artificial tubal blockage are options if your family is complete. Before embarking on either of these alternatives, you will need counselling and a full explanation of the techniques used.

Postnatal exercise

As soon as your baby is born, you can begin gentle exercises to help you recover from birth and get back into shape. Exercising after birth is not about trying to fit into your pre-pregnancy clothes. Postnatal exercise is about looking after yourself. It's okay to take a little time for yourself. Exercise after birth provides you with both positive physical and emotional benefits.

You can begin some of these exercises from the first day after birth, but it can take six months to a year to completely regain your pre-baby figure. You can breastfeed to help lose the extra weight gained in pregnancy, and after a while, try walking, swimming, pilates or yoga.

> If you've had a caesarean birth, you can start doing pelvic floor exercises straight away. You can begin with deep abdominal muscle strengthening exercises in the first few days following birth, followed by pelvic tilt (see next section). Delay doing stronger abdominal exercises until your incision has healed or if you've been given the okay by a health professional.

Abdominal muscle separation

Before beginning more strenuous abdominal exercises, check that the abdominal muscles between the lower ribs and the pubic bone have come together. These muscles have to stretch to allow the baby to grow, and after the birth, remain slightly apart. It would help if you waited until you can only insert the tips of two fingers in the space between them while you raise your head from the pillow. Reversal of abdominal separation takes about eight weeks following the birth.

> **If you have four fingers or more abdominal separation, consult a health professional specialising in post-birth recovery.**

Pelvic floor exercises

These can be started right after birth and are especially important because pelvic floor muscles stretch considerably during birth. If you have stitches or haemorrhoids, exercise to the point of discomfort.

Doing these exercises will help reduce swelling and restore the supportive muscles underneath, helpful aids to increasing comfort. The pelvic floor exercises are the same as those practised in pregnancy; see page 14 for details.

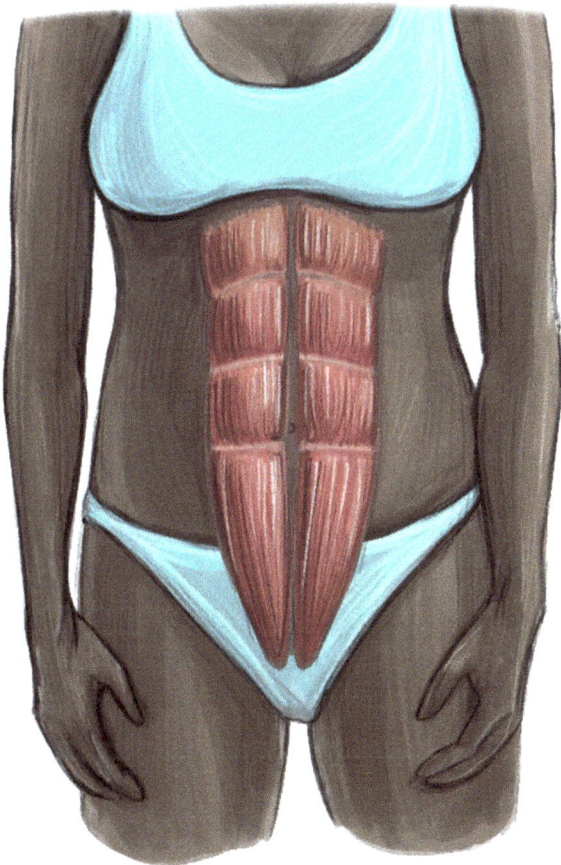

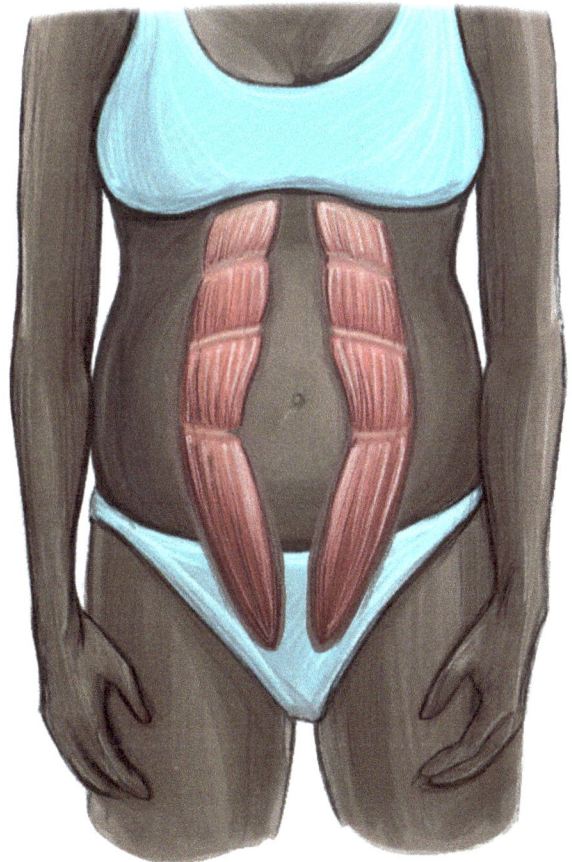

Each time you pick the baby up, cough or have to lift anything, tighten the pelvic floor and lower abdominal muscles first. It takes time for the pelvic floor muscles to recover their former strength.

Deep abdominal muscle strengthening

The first step is to engage the deepest muscle in the stomach, which acts like a corset. Deep abdominal muscles support your torso, allow movement and hold your organs in place.

Find a comfortable position – side-lying or lying on your back are excellent positions to start. Let your tummy sag and breathe in gently. As you breathe out, tighten your pelvic floor and, at the same time, draw in the lower part of your stomach towards your spine and hold for a few seconds, then relax. As you get stronger, hold for longer. The aim is to hold for ten seconds and repeat ten times eventually. Ideally, do this exercise three times a day.

You should be able to talk and breathe while doing this exercise, with no breath-holding. As you get stronger, you can do this exercise sitting or standing.

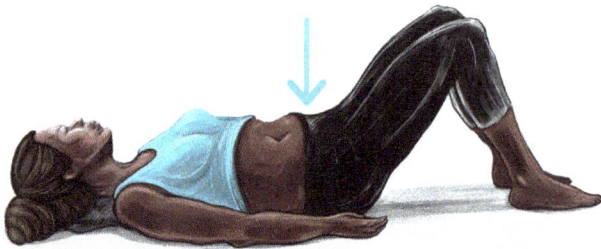

Once you can comfortably do this exercise, you can begin the pelvic tilt and progress to head lifts, as your comfort level dictates.

If you notice any bulging or peaking of your abdominal muscles while doing any of the following exercises, stop and return to deep abdominal muscle strengthening and seek advice from a specialist postnatal manual therapist.

> **If you notice any bulging or peaking of your abdominal muscles while doing any of the following exercises, stop and return to deep abdominal muscle strengthening and seek advice from a specialist postnatal manual therapist.**

Pelvic tilt

The pelvic tilt is a simple exercise that will help relieve backache and improve abdominal strength. Lie on your back and tighten your abdominal muscles as you flatten your lower spine against the floor and release. Repeat several times in succession.

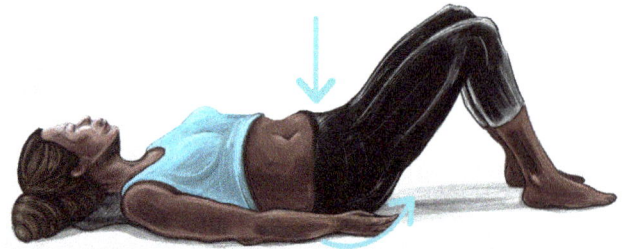

> **Don't do the following exercises if you have abdominal separation (unless under the guidance of a health professional).**

Head lift

The following exercise to progress to is the head lift. Rest with your head on a pillow, perform the pelvic tilt, squeeze your pelvic floor muscles and lift your head and hold for three seconds, lower and then relax. Repeat the head lift up to ten times in a row. Ideally, do a set three times per day.

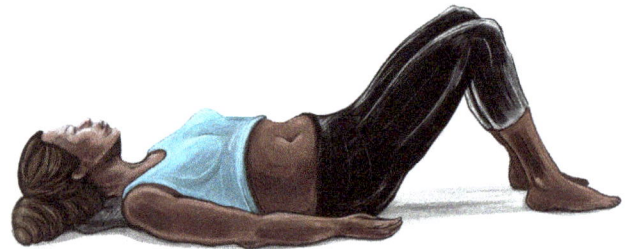

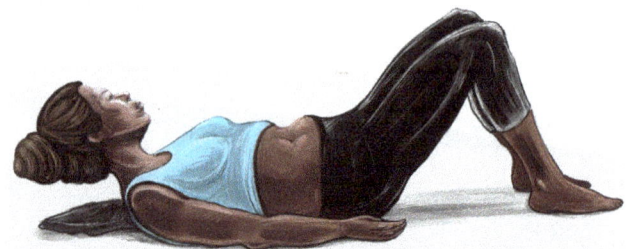

Side reaching

Raise your head and shoulders to reach across your body to the outside of one knee. Hold briefly, then release. Do the opposite side, breathing out as you reach up and in as you release.

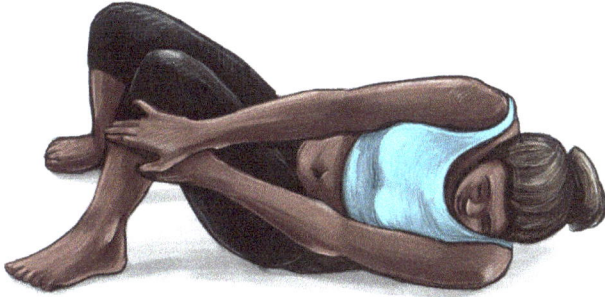

Lay down with your knees bent and your feet flat on the floor. Sit your baby on your lap with their back supported on your thighs. Then sit up, lifting your shoulders and head to talk to your baby.

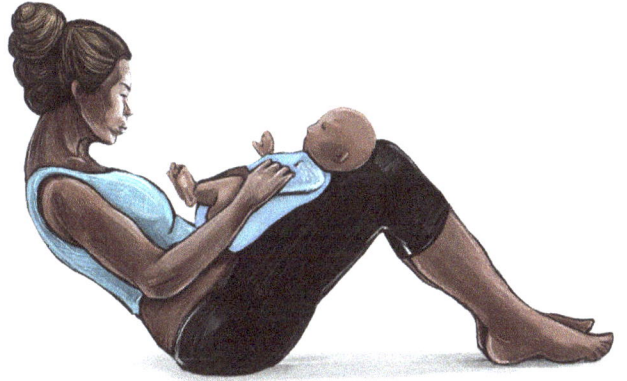

Exercising with your baby

When you are ready for more vigorous exercise, include your baby. It's fun for you both and can form part of your daily playtime.

Lay your baby along your legs. Tighten your buttocks and pelvic floor and lift your hips slowly until they form a straight line with your back and shoulders. Unroll gradually.

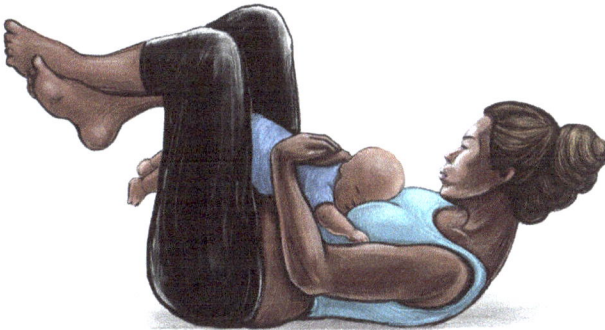

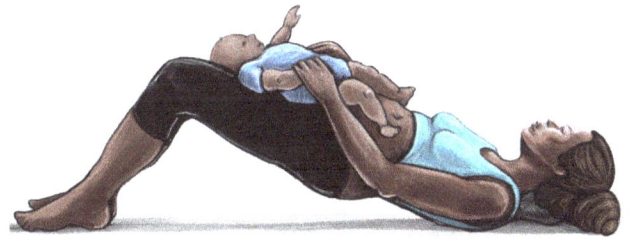

Lay your baby on your tummy and raise your head and shoulders while bringing your knees to your chest. Rest with your feet off the floor. Repeat up to ten times. When you have finished, lower one foot first, then the other.

Lay your baby on the floor. Starting on hands and knees, extend one arm and the opposite leg, no higher than the hip level. Change over, and exercise the other arm and leg.

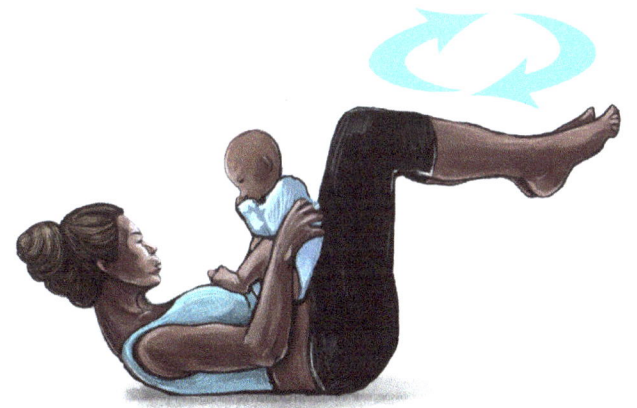

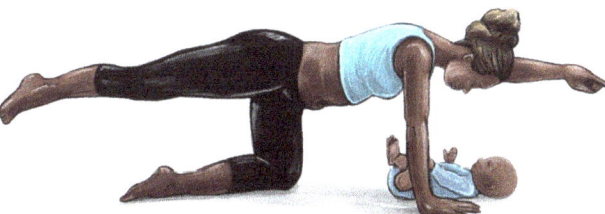

Next, sit your baby on your pubic bone supported by your legs. Hold on to your baby's chest as you circle around with your legs. Raise your head and shoulders at the same time.

Notes

www.ingramcontent.com/pod-product-compliance
Lightning Source LLC
Chambersburg PA
CBHW042347030426
42335CB00031B/3489